The Handbook of
Early Stuttering Intervention

D1417837

The Handbook of Early Stuttering Intervention

Edited by

Mark Onslow
Ann Packman

Australian Stuttering Research Centre
The University of Sydney

SINGULAR PUBLISHING GROUP, INC.
SAN DIEGO · LONDON

Singular Publishing Group, Inc.
401 West "A" Street, Suite 325
San Diego, California 92101-7904

Singular Publishing Ltd.
19 Compton Terrace
London, N1 2UN, UK

Singular Publishing Group, Inc., publishes textbooks, clinical manuals, clinical reference books, journals, videos, and multimedia materials on speech-language pathology, audiology, otorhinolaryngology, special education, early childhood, aging, occupational therapy, physical therapy, rehabilitation, counseling, mental health, and voice. For your convenience, our entire catalog can be accessed on our website at *http://www.singpub.com.* Our mission to provide you with materials to meet the daily challenges of the ever-changing health care/educational environment will remain on course if we are in touch with you. In that spirit, we welcome your feedback on our products. Please telephone (**1-800-521-8545**), fax (**1-800-774-8398**), or e-mail (*singpub@singpub.com*) your comments and requests to us.

Typeset in 10/12 Bookman by So Cal Graphics
Printed in the United States of America by Bang Printing

Library of Congress Cataloging-in-Publication Data

The handbook of early stuttering intervention/edited by Mark Onslow
     and Ann Packman.
          p.   cm.
     Includes bibliographical references and index.
     ISBN 1–56593–970–0
     1. Stuttering in children—Treatment—Handbooks, manuals, etc.
  2. Speech therapy for children—Handbooks, manuals, etc.
  I. Onslow, Mark.   II. Packman, Ann.
     [DNLM: 1. Stuttering—in infancy & childhood.   2. Stuttering-
  -therapy.   WM 475 H2358 1999]
  RJ496.S8H36   1999
  618.92'855—dc21
  DNLM/DLC
  for Library of Congress   98–55683
                                                                   CIP

Contents

Preface

The impetus to assemble this book was the rapid proliferation of documented treatment procedures for stuttering in preschool children. In recent years, we have found it quite a task to keep an overview of theoretical and empirical developments in this important field of speech-language pathology, and our main purpose in the compilation of chapters that follow is to make it a little easier for others to do so. We are not completely sure who all of those others may be, but certainly they would include students and generalist clinicians who wish to acquire an overview of this clinical field as it stands in 1999. Perhaps those with specialist knowledge will find value also in the collection in one place of the work of so many who are experts in this pursuit, and will be intrigued by the summary of our wise and level-headed commentator, Dr Attanasio. Perhaps those seeking out controversy will be drawn also to what our contributors have put before us. Historically, the issue of what to do with children who begin to stutter has attracted many different views, and the contents of this book show things to be much the same. Clearly, that is how it will be for some time. If nothing else, this text is a document of the state of play in 1999.

Early in 1998 we began to solicit contributions to this project. Some of our contributors have developed treatments exclusively for preschool children who stutter; others developed their treatments for a wider age range. For the latter contributors, we asked that they tailor their contributions to describe what their programs offer for preschoolers. We are delighted to have obtained contributions from so many authorities of the day. The publication of their work, so soon in 1999, is a testament to their diligence as authors, the firm insistence of Marie Linvill at Singular and the eagle eye of Joan Rosenthal.

We believe that, collectively, the contributors of this text convey that there is uncertainty in our field about how to help children who begin to stutter in their first years of life. That is how it should be, for, in our judgment at least, we are a long way

preschool focus only

from knowing the most effective and efficient way to manage early stuttering. Perhaps, somewhere in what follows, one of our contributors has written something which can lead us to that knowledge. Perhaps it will be a student who reads the work of our contributors and is inspired to work at the problem, and who ultimately develops effective and efficient treatment methods for stuttering in early childhood. That would be the best outcome of our efforts.

Contributors

Joseph S. Attanasio, Ph.D.
Department of
 Communication Sciences
 and Disorders
Montclair State University
Upper Montclair, New Jersey
USA

Edward G. Conture, Ph.D.
Vanderbilt Bill Wilkerson
 Center for Otolaryngology
 and Communication
 Sciences and Disorders
Vanderbilt University
Nashville, Tennessee
USA

**Sheryl Ridener Gottwald,
 Ph.D.**
New England Center for
 Speech-Language Services
Bedford, New Hampshire
USA

Hugo H. Gregory, Ph.D.
Professor Emeritus
Department of
 Communication Sciences
 and Disorders
Northwestern University
Evanston, Illinois
USA

**Elisabeth Harrison,
 B.App.Sc. (Sp Path)**
Senior Speech Pathologist,
 Stuttering Unit
Bankstown Health Service
Bankstown, New South Wales
Australia

Michelle Lincoln, Ph.D.
School of Communication
 Sciences and Disorders
The University of Sydney
Lidcombe, New South Wales
Australia

Kenneth S. Melnick
Vanderbilt University
Nashville, Tennesse

Mark Onslow, Ph.D.
Director, Australian
 Stuttering Research Centre
Associate Professor, The
 University of Sydney
Lidcombe, New South Wales
Australia

Ann Packman, Ph.D.
Australian Stuttering
 Research Centre
The University of Sydney
Lidcombe, New South Wales
Australia

Rebekah H. Pindzola, Ph.D.
Professor, Department of
   Communication Disorders
Associate Dean, College of
   Liberal Arts
Auburn University
Auburn, Alabama
USA

Glyndon Riley, Ph.D.
Executive Director, Center for
   Children Who Stutter
California State University
Fullerton, California
USA

Jeanna Riley, Ph.D.
Director, Rileys Speech and
   Language Institute
Tustin, California
USA

Charles M. Runyan, Ph.D.
Department of Speech
   Pathology and Audiology
James Madison University
Harrisonburg, Virginia
USA

**Sara Elizabeth Runyan,
   Ph.D.**
Department of Speech
   Pathology and Audiology
James Madison University
Harrisonburg, Virginia
USA

**Barbara Van Kirk Ryan,
   Ph.D.**
Communicative Disorders
   Department
California State University
Long Beach, California
USA

Bruce P. Ryan, Ph.D.
Communicative Disorders
   Department
California State University
Long Beach, California
USA

**C. Woodruff Starkweather,
   Ph.D.**
Temple University
Philadelphia, Pennsylvania
USA

Issues in the Treatment of Early Stuttering

ANN PACKMAN
MARK ONSLOW

It is now widely agreed that treating stuttering in early childhood is preferable to waiting until the disorder is more established and less tractable. One testament to this is the proliferation, over the last decade or so, of reports of treatments for children who start to stutter. Much of this recent interest in treating stuttering in young children can be attributed to the waning popularity of Wendell Johnson's view that drawing attention to the speech of these children will worsen their stuttering. The publication of a text on early intervention by Prins and Ingham (1983) signified unequivocally that prominent clinicians no longer regarded Johnson's view as "perceived wisdom."

This reversal in position on the management of early stuttering has widespread ramifications. On the positive side, there is no longer a conspiracy of silence about early stuttering (Rustin & Cook, 1995); that is, children need no longer believe that stuttering is so awful that no one will talk about it. And, of course, many children are now being protected by early intervention from a lifetime of stuttering. However, we must not lose sight of the fact that treatments now typically draw the attention of young children who stutter to their speech, and so children are now confronting their stuttering at an earlier age. Thus, if treatment is unsuccessful, treatment failure will occur far earlier than before, and the adult client with a long history of unsatisfactory treatment is already an all too common presentation (Gregory & Hill, 1993). Parents and sometimes entire families may be actively included in the treatment process, which may be quite time consuming and even stressful. In short, although it is no longer thought that drawing attention to stuttering in young children will necessarily make the condition worse, clinicians need to carefully consider the impact of this "new wave" of treatments on children and their families in both the short and the long term.

Other issues about the implementation of treatment for early stuttering are now being discussed in the literature. The most pressing are (a) whether to treat all children who stutter, (b) when to implement treatment, and (c) what treatment to use. These issues are more complex with young children than they are with adolescents and adults, because many children who start to stutter will recover without treatment. In this chapter, we overview the most salient of these issues. We have decided to couch them in the form of questions; questions that clinicians typically ask themselves and, indeed, that are typically asked of them by parents, other professionals, and those who fund treatment. We have identified six questions. It is not our intention to canvass these issues fully here, nor are we in a position to provide definitive answers to these questions. Rather, we raise these issues so that readers will have a context in which to consider the treatments presented in the following chapters.

QUESTIONS ABOUT TREATMENT

Question 1: How Does a Clinician Know That a Child Is Stuttering?

The diagnosis of stuttering in young children is a vexed question in the literature. The most commonly discussed issue—distinguishing between stuttering and normal disfluency—has engaged scholars and theoreticians for decades. In practice, however, deciding whether a child is stuttering is usually quite straightforward. Children are normally brought to a clinic because a parent or parents think they are stuttering and in most cases the diagnosis of stuttering is not problematic. On a perceptual level alone, it is usually clear whether a child's speech contains sufficient aberrant speech behaviors to warrant a diagnosis of stuttering. In other words, in most instances a clinician or student clinician who has had reasonable exposure to stuttering and to the speech and language of normally developing preschool children will have little difficulty deciding that a child is stuttering.

Nonetheless, for this type of perceptual diagnosis, consensus between two clinicians and a parent, and possibly another important person in the child's life, is usually sought before making a definite pronouncement that a child is stuttering (J. C. Ingham, 1993; Onslow, 1992).

However, there are some children whose disfluencies are fleeting and infrequent and for whom diagnosing stuttering is more difficult. Parents may report the occurrence outside the clinic of speech disruptions that are clearly stuttering, but the child fails to demonstrate them in the clinic. Further, stuttering in young children may appear, disappear, and appear again over a period of weeks or months. In short, although a positive identification of stuttering is clear-cut in most cases, negative identification—deciding that a child is not stuttering—may be more difficult. In such cases, a period of monitoring is usually recommended until consensus is reached on either a positive or negative identification (Onslow, 1992).

The commonly used alternative to the consensus diagnosis is a behavioral diagnosis. This is based on an analysis of disfluencies and typically involves, among other things, identifying all of a child's speech disruptions and deciding, according to objective criteria, whether the child is stuttering, not stuttering, or displaying borderline stuttering. A number of protocols and behavioral checklists are available for this purpose (for a review see Gordon & Luper, 1993).

An issue closely related to diagnosing stuttering is how to decide whether individual speech disruptions are stutters. Again, there are two somewhat polarized positions. One advocates a perceptual procedure, whereby a categorical judgment is made for each disfluency as to whether it is a stutter or not. Such judgments are involved in frequency measures of stuttering, for example, percent syllables stuttered. Categorical judgments of stuttered/not stuttered are also involved in interval measures of stuttering (see Cordes & Ingham, 1995). Proponents of the second position advocate behavioral identification, where the topography of each disfluency determines how it will be categorized according to disfluency taxonomies such as Stuttering-Like/Other (Yairi & Ambrose, 1992), More Typical/Less Typical and More Usual/More Unusual (Gregory & Hill, 1993), and Between/Within Word (Conture, 1990). This process does not involve judging whether a disfluency is stuttered or not and has provided the context for the idea that normal children sometimes stutter. This notion is difficult to reconcile semantically if the behaviors that constitute stuttering are considered to be pathological.

As with most issues pertaining to young children, then, diagnosing stuttering is not clear-cut, and there is no "correct" way to do it. Consequently, many clinicians use a combination of identification and diagnostic procedures. For example, in accepting children for the Illinois Early Childhood Stuttering Project, Yairi and colleagues rely on (a) parental and clinician agreement that the child is stuttering, (b) a Stuttering-Like Disfluency frequency of three or more per hundred syllables, and (c) above 2 on an 8-point stuttering severity scale (Yairi & Ambrose, 1992).

One unresolved issue in diagnosing stuttering concerns the nature of certain disfluency types. It has been reported many times that the first signs of stuttering are repetitions of syllables and that parents almost always say that this is the first thing that alerted them to the possibility that their child might be stuttering (see Bloodstein, 1995). It was previously thought that these repetitions were followed gradually by the other speech disruptions that have come to be associated with more advanced or secondary stuttering, such as prolongations and blocks, and it is widely believed that these more effortful speech behaviors are a reaction to or an attempt to avoid the original repetitions.

It is now known, however, that more effortful stuttering involving fixed postures may be present very soon after the onset of stuttering (see Yairi, 1997) and it is not at all clear, despite a long-standing belief, that these behaviors constitute attempts to avoid repetitions. These so-called secondary behaviors may simply be another form of stuttering—another manifestation of the difficulty the child is having in mobilizing the speech mechanism appropriately. The idea that prolongations and blocks are a reaction to repetitions is intuitively appealing but not necessarily correct (see Packman & Onslow, 1998a).

In any event, there is still no consensus about whether syllable repetitions are truly stuttering. Yairi includes single-syllable repetitions (including single-syllable word repetitions) in his Stuttering-Like Disfluencies category; however, Conture (1990) suggests that single-syllable word repetitions may reflect "pure expressive language delays" (p. 60) rather than stuttering. Starkweather (1997) also does not consider whole-word and whole-syllable repetitions to be stuttering, but suggests that stuttering is "the extraneous effort, the reactions, and the struggles that can develop in response to those disfluencies" (p. 79). On the other hand, Starkweather does not believe that the repetitions that are thought to characterize the onset of stuttering are normal either.

Thus, the issue is whether a child who only repeats syllables, such as "I-I-I-I-I-wanna juice, Mummy," is indeed stuttering. This seems to be largely a matter of semantics intertwined with questions about the nature and course of stuttering discussed above, and from a behavioral perspective at least, it makes little sense *not* to regard these syllable repetitions as stuttering, because syllable repetitions are widely regarded as part of the disorder.

So, after decades of research and discussion, scholars and researchers still do not agree on the nature of early stuttering and how to identify, describe, and categorize it (Packman & Onslow, 1998a). Finding some consensus on these issues would be helpful because it would contribute to more effective communication about stuttering and its treatment. Until that time, however, clinicians will presumably choose the diagnostic methods with which they are most comfortable.

Question 2: Is Treatment for Early Stuttering Effective?

Although there are many reports of effective treatments for young children who stutter, it is also known that many of these children will recover without professional intervention (Andrews, 1984; Yairi & Ambrose, 1992). Thus, it can be argued that treatments reported to be effective with these children are in some cases simply reflecting the natural recovery process.

There are two related but distinct issues to address here (see Packman & Onslow, 1998b). The first is whether treatment is more effective than natural (spontaneous) recovery, *in the long run*. In other words, if treated children were compared after many years with untreated children, would more children in the treated group be stutter-free?

At present, we do not know the answer to this question because the necessary research has not been done. Such research would require withholding treatment from a group of children until the natural recovery process is complete, a process that Yairi and Ambrose (1992) suggested may take more than 2 years. Yet parents seek treatment for their children for many reasons, not the least of which is that they and/or their child are frustrated or distressed about the stuttering. Hence, they are unlikely to be willing to forego treatment for such a long period and may seek treatment elsewhere. Onslow and colleagues found this to be the case some years ago (see Onslow, Andrews, & Lincoln, 1994) when they found that they could not convince parents to withhold treatment from their children in the cause of science.

This may become less of a problem if it turns out that delaying treatment for some time—within the preschool years—may not worsen the ultimate outcome (see Onslow, Harrison, Jones, & Packman, 1998).

The second issue relating to the effectiveness of treatment is whether treatment has an *immediate* impact on the natural course of the child's stuttering. That is, does the child stop stuttering when the treatment is given, and is that improvement attributable to the treatment and not to some other factor? In our view, this is a much more important question for clinicians than a statistical question about the speech performance of groups of children in the long term. For the sake of accountability, clinicians want to know that when they introduce treatment there are immediate and documentable benefits for the child and family.

Although there are numerous reports in the literature of the benefits of treatment for early stuttering, few are supported by evidence of effectiveness (Cordes, 1998) and even treatments that report outcome data must be considered to be only in the preliminary stages of development. For example, the work of Onslow and colleagues on evaluation of the Lidcombe Program is at an early stage, the research having been conducted on volunteers, under relatively ideal conditions and without randomly selected control groups (Onslow, 1998).

Question 3: Which Children Should a Clinician Treat and When?

Natural recovery poses a number of dilemmas for clinicians who are charged with managing young children who stutter. For example, while parents are usually concerned about their child's stuttering, it can be argued that routinely treating every child is overservicing because in the long run some portion of these children will recover without treatment. Thus, it has been suggested that young children who come to a clinic could be monitored until they have been stuttering for 1 or 2 years, to allow natural recovery to occur (Curlee & Yairi, 1997). However, this means that clinicians would leave young children to stutter when effective treatments are available. Although that may not be a problem for children who start to recover during that time, for children who do not recover, treatment will have been postponed much longer than necessary. We do not yet know whether time since onset influences tractability or responsiveness to treatment (Ingham &

Cordes, 1998a), although, as we mentioned earlier, this may not be the case for children participating in the Lidcombe Program (Onslow et al., 1998).

It is by no means clear, either, that waiting for up 2 years before implementing treatment is without consequences for the child and family. For example, we simply do not know the effects on a child's social, emotional, cognitive, and linguistic development of allowing stuttering to continue in the hope that the child will recover naturally.

In any event, Curlee and Yairi (1997) tempered their advice to monitor stuttering by saying that treatment should be implemented earlier if children are reacting negatively to their stuttering, if the parents want them treated, if they are 5 years or older, or if they have other communication problems. We agree with these recommendations. For it would be bordering on unethical not to treat children who are having difficulty communicating and who are frustrated or distressed about their stuttering when effective treatments are available. Nor would a clinician feel comfortable advising parents who are concerned about their child's stuttering, perhaps because they themselves stutter, to adopt the "wait and hope" approach. Of course, many parents are reassured when told that their child may recover naturally and that effective treatments are available and are prepared to wait and see, but many are not.

One action that clinicians can take when children come to the clinic is to investigate whether they are already in the recovery process. This can be done by actively monitoring the child's stuttering for some period (see Ingham & Riley, 1998). For example, parents could mail tape recordings of their child's speech to the clinician every month. If stuttering is not decreasing over some period, perhaps a few months, then the clinician can introduce treatment and have some confidence that the changes that occur are attributable to the treatment and not to natural factors (see Ingham & Riley, 1998). This procedure does not mean that a child with recent onset might not have recovered anyway at a later time, since natural recovery[1] may take 2 years or even longer in some cases. But clinicians can be more confident in claiming a cause-effect relationship between the treatment and the improvement.

---

[1] We prefer the term "natural recovery," even though it is less widely used than "spontaneous recovery," because it implies that there are factors in nature responsible for such recovery. For a discussion of this issue see Finn (1998) and R. J. Ingham (1983).

Of course, information that would help identify children who are more likely to recover naturally would be of enormous value here, because it would allow clinicians to intervene early with children who are not going to recover naturally. What is known about factors that predict whether children will recover naturally from stuttering or whether they will continue to stutter into adulthood? Considerable information about such factors is emanating from the Illinois Early Childhood Stuttering Project, which is studying the natural course of stuttering in the general population. Children are recruited within 1 year of onset and monitored for some years, after which they are allocated to either the "recovered" or the "persistent" group. According to the findings of the Illinois project, children whose stuttering recovers naturally (a) are likely to have started stuttering 5 to 8 months earlier than other children, (b) tend to have relatives who have recovered naturally from stuttering, and (c) are likely to be female. Also, because most recovery has occurred by 2 years postonset (Yairi & Ambrose, 1992), the longer a child has been stuttering the less likely the child is to recover without formal treatment.

The Illinois project has also identified factors that do not appear to be associated with recovery and persistence. First, stuttering severity apparently does not predict natural recovery. Second, measures of spontaneous language such as mean length of utterance, number of different words, and number of total words do not predict recovery (Watkins & Yairi, 1997). Third, although there is a weak relationship between superior phonological development and natural recovery. (Yairi, Ambrose, Paden, & Throneburg, 1996) this relationship does not appear to be clinically useful.

In the Illinois project, factors identified as associated with recovery or persistence, and factors identified as not associated with recovery or persistence, are statistically derived. In other words, findings must be considered in terms of probability. Identifying a factor that predicts natural recovery does not guarantee recovery in every case (Bernstein Ratner, 1997; Packman & Onslow, 1998b), and clinicians can never say to a parent with 100% certainty that their child will or will not recover without treatment. For example, while most girls recover spontaneously, we still cannot say in advance *which* girls will recover. We only know that a girl has a much better chance of recovering without treatment than a boy.

Information about natural recovery generated by the Illinois project can be applied in clinical practice in a risk analysis (Zebrowski, 1997). On the one hand, a clinician may choose not to immediately treat a girl who has been stuttering for only a few months and who has a family history of recovery, because she has a good chance of recovering naturally. On the other hand, a boy who has been stuttering for more than a year and whose father stutters would be considered at higher risk of continuing to stutter and would be a more pressing candidate for treatment. And if such a boy had been stuttering for 2 years the likelihood of recovery would be even lower, and immediate treatment would be a priority.

In summary, given our current understanding of early stuttering, there are no hard and fast rules about whether to treat a particular stuttering child who comes to the clinic (Packman & Lincoln, 1998). Although scientifically established predictor factors may be taken into account, they cannot, on their own, lead the clinician to the "correct" decision about whether to intervene with a particular child. In the absence of clear guidelines, then, clinicians will consider the particular circumstances surrounding each child. The distress of a child and/or a parent is surely sufficient grounds for intervening quickly. Such a decision will not be based on science but rather will depend on the clinician's judgment about the welfare of the child.

Question 4: How Does a Clinician Decide Which Treatment to Use?

At first glance the choice of treatments for early stuttering may seem a bewildering one, and indeed the chapters in this book illustrate the variety of treatment approaches available to clinicians. A number of factors will be at work as clinicians decide which treatment to use. For example, many will be attracted in the first instance to a treatment that is congruent with their views on the nature of stuttering and their theoretical position on what causes it. These views are likely to have been formed, in part, by the views and preferences of mentors, supervisors, or even the institutions or organizations in which people work. Cultural factors may also play a part. For example, there are considerable differences across countries and cultures in views about stuttering and how it should be managed (Attanasio, Onslow, & Packman, 1996). Following are some ways of categorizing treatment approaches that might provide a useful background to the treatments presented in this text. We present five taxonomies, or ways of describing treatments:

5 Tx taxonomies

1. Treatments may involve (a) *environmental change*, which is the alteration of aspects of the family environment; (b) *speech pattern change*, which aims to alter the child's and/or the parental speech patterns; (c) *operant procedures*, which arrange contingencies for stuttered and stutter-free speech; or (d) *linguistic simplification procedures*, which reduce the linguistic complexity of the child's utterances.
2. Treatments may be *direct* or *indirect*, according to whether they draw attention to the child's speech.
3. Treatments may be *programmed* (systematic), progressing in predetermined stages or steps, or they may be *nonprogrammed*, in that the principles of treatment are only loosely prescribed and clinicians are free to make ad hoc decisions about the conduct of the treatment as it progresses.
4. Treatments may be categorized according to their derivation. For example, some treatments have a *theoretical* base, in that the therapy is derived from a particular view of the cause and/or nature of stuttering; other treatments are *atheoretical* and driven solely by data.
5. Treatments may be *standardized*, in that each child receives more or less the same procedure, or they may be highly *individualized*, in that a different treatment regimen is implemented for each child.

Of course, most treatments consist of a "package" of procedures and do not fit clearly into one or other of the categories included in these five taxonomies. Nonetheless, the taxonomies provide a way of ascertaining the primary focus of a treatment.

However, the most important factor to consider in deciding which treatment to use is probably its efficacy (Ingham & Cordes, 1998b), for clinicians do not want to offer a treatment that does not work. This perspective is consistent with the move to evidence-based medicine, where practitioners are expected to provide treatments that have empirical support.

Question 5: How Can a Clinician Verify That a Treatment is Working?

The obvious answer to this question is to measure change in the children who receive the treatment. However, exactly what to measure depends on the desired outcome of the treatment. Clearly, a desirable outcome with preschool children who stutter is that they stop stuttering, and there are well-established means using objective measures of stuttering to demonstrate such an outcome (e.g., see Ingham & Riley, 1998). However, our profession is moving towards instituting assessments of functional outcomes, such as scaling a child's eagerness to communicate in various situations (see Baum, 1998; Cordes, Finn, Ingham, & Packman, 1998; Shenker, Kully, & Meltzer, 1998). The value of functional outcome measures is yet to be determined with young children who stutter, because such measures are likely to be functionally related to the level of the child's stuttering. In our experience, parents almost always report that children are more effective and enthusiastic communicators once the stuttering is gone.

Ingham and Cordes (1998b) described a 3-factor model for stuttering outcome research that can, with minimal alteration, be used as a basis for measuring effectiveness in the clinic. First, to conform to this model, children should be actively monitored for a considerable time after the intensive stage of treatment to ensure that the benefits of treatment are maintained. As mentioned earlier, stuttering in young children may vary considerably across time, sometimes disappearing and reappearing over days or weeks; thus, one measure at the end of treatment showing that a child is not stuttering is not sufficient to demonstrate the effectiveness of the treatment in the long term. Second, stuttering should be monitored outside the clinic as well as inside the clinic, because speech performance in the two situations may be quite different. It cannot be assumed that children no longer stutter in everyday situations simply because they are not stuttering in the clinic. Third, measures of stuttering used to show effectiveness should be reliable.

Question 6: How Long Will Treatment Take?

The current enthusiasm for treating early stuttering has been sustained by increasing knowledge that effective treatment is less time-consuming for preschool children than it is for adults (see Onslow, 1996). That notwithstanding, clinicians need to be able to give parents an estimate of how long treatment might be expected to take.

Parents are not the only stakeholders here. Funding bodies also want this information. The funding of the delivery of speech-language pathology services varies across countries, and even within countries. For example, such services may be funded by a government department or agency, a managed care organization, or through health insurance companies. In these times of ever decreasing health care budgets, the organizations that pay for the delivery of speech-language pathology services continue to demand documentation not only of the effectiveness of treatment but also of its efficiency. In other words, a priority for funding bodies is that more services be provided with fewer resources. In the case of treatment for early stuttering, these resources are clinical hours. This focus puts considerable pressure on clinicians to account for the hours spent treating young children who stutter.

Although efficiency is typically the most important factor for funding bodies, it is not the only factor that clinicians take into consideration when planning their services. Their primary responsibility is a duty of care to their clients. Hewat and Wilson (1998) provided a model for understanding the difficult task faced by clinicians in balancing efficiency, which is demanded from managers and funding bodies, with equity and quality, which are important from the perspective of their clients. Equity implies fairness or justice both in access to services and in service delivery across groups in the community, whereas quality includes such factors as the effectiveness and acceptability of treatments, and consumer satisfaction. Thus, continual pressure from funding bodies on clinicians to be efficient has the potential to lead to a "trade-off" of equity and quality. Yet, from the clinician's perspective, reducing treatment time is not acceptable if the treatment is not also fair, effective, and acceptable.

Apart from accountability to funding bodies, knowledge about likely treatment time can also be used profitably in the treatment process itself. For example, if clinicians know the average time taken to eliminate stuttering with a particular treatment, then they can check the clinical progress of each client. This principle can apply to a treatment program or to a component of a treatment program. Consider, for example, a situation in which a child has made only modest progress in treatment but treatment has already consumed well over the average number of hours. This would identify the problematic status of that child and should prompt an inquiry into the reasons for such slow progress.

The point of all this is that, more and more, clinicians need benchmark information from the developers of treatment programs about how long treatment is likely to take. Such data will require large numbers of subjects to provide reliable group data. At the same time, information can be gathered about factors that influence treatment time. Such factors, if they are mutable, might be used for the purposes of clinic time management. For example, if younger children take fewer clinical hours to treat, then it may be more efficient to adopt a policy of intervening as soon as possible after onset, although, of course, the value of this approach would need to be weighed against the knowledge that some clinical hours will be saved by delaying treatment and allowing natural recovery to occur in some children. Such considerations represent just one more dilemma facing clinicians who treat young children who start to stutter. On the other hand, knowing that stuttering severity influences treatment time will contribute little to increasing clinical efficiency, because severity of stuttering is, in this context, immutable.

CONCLUSION

In introducing this text, we noted a strong trend in our profession toward the treatment of stuttering in the preschool years. This trend is characterized by diverse treatment methods and a growing body of empirical support for their effectiveness. We also identified a number of related issues that face clinicians in their everyday workplace. Those issues include how to diagnose stuttering, whether treatment has a positive impact on the natural course of the disorder, whether to treat all children and when to intervene with those who are treated, which treatment to use, and how long treatment can be expected to take. Most of these issues are only at the threshold of resolution, and all we have done here is highlight them and put them on record. Perhaps in an introduction to a future edition of this book, there will be many more answers to the questions we have raised.

REFERENCES

Andrews, G. (1984). Epidemiology of stuttering. In R. F. Curlee & W. H. Perkins (Eds.), *Nature and treatment of stuttering: New directions* (pp. 1–12). San Diego, CA: College-Hill Press.

Attanasio, J. S., Onslow, M., & Packman, A. (1996). Australian and United States perspectives on stuttering in preschool children. *Australian Journal of Human Communication Disorders*, 24, 55–61.

Baum, H. M. (1998, August). Response from Herbert Baum, *Fluency and Fluency Disorders*, p. 9.

Bernstein Ratner, N. (1997). Leaving Las Vegas: Clinical odds and individual outcomes. *American Journal of Speech-Language Pathology, 6*(2), 29–33.

Bloodstein, O. (1995). *A handbook of stuttering* (5th ed.). San Diego, CA: Singular Publishing Group.

Conture, E. G. (1990). *Stuttering* (2nd ed.). Englewood Cliffs, NJ: Prentice-Hall.

Cordes, A. (1998). Current status of the stuttering treatment literature. In A. K. Cordes & R. J. Ingham (Eds.), *Treatment efficacy for stuttering: A search for empirical bases* (pp. 117–144). San Diego, CA. Singular Publishing Group.

Cordes, A., Finn, P., Ingham, R. J., & Packman, A. C. (1998, August). Reflections on the 1998 Division 4 meeting. *Fluency and Fluency Disorders*, pp. 7–9.

Cordes, A. K., & Ingham, R. J. (1995). Judgments of stuttered and nonstuttered intervals by recognized authorities in stuttering research. *Journal of Speech and Hearing Research, 38*, 33–41.

Curlee, R. F., & Yairi, E. (1997). Early intervention with early childhood stuttering: A critical examination of the data. *Americal Journal of Speech-Language Pathology, 6*(2), 8–18.

Finn, P. (1998). Recovery without treatment: A review of conceptual and methodological considerations across disciplines. In A. K. Cordes & R. J. Ingham (Eds.), *Treatment efficacy for stuttering: A search for empirical bases* (pp. 3–25). San Diego, CA: Singular Publishing Group.

Gordon, P. A., & Luper, H. L. (1993). The early identification of stuttering. I: Protocols. *American Journal of Speech-Language Pathology, 2*, 43–53.

Gregory, H. H., & Hill, D. (1993). Differential evaluation—Different therapy for stuttering children. In R. F. Curlee (Ed.), *Stuttering and related disorders of fluency* (pp. 23–44). New York: Thieme Medical Publishers.

Hewat, S., & Wilson, L. (1998). Balancing the efficiency, equity, and quality of a service. *Advances in Speech Language Pathology* (in press).

Ingham, J. C. (1993). Behavioral treatment of stuttering children. In R. F. Curlee (Ed.), *Stuttering and related disorders of fluency* (pp. 68–89). New York: Thieme Medical Publishers.

Ingham, J. C., & Riley, G. (1998). Guidelines for documentation of treatment efficacy for young children who stutter. *Journal of Speech, Language and Hearing Research, 41*, 753–770.

Ingham, R. J. (1983). Spontaneous remission of stuttering: When will the emperor realize he has no clothes on? In D. Prins & R. J. Ingham (Eds.), *Treatment of early stuttering in early childhood: Methods and issues* (pp. 113–140). San Diego, CA: College-Hill Press.

Ingham, R. J., & Cordes, A. K. (1998a). Treatment decisions for young children who stutter: Further concerns and complexities. *American Journal of Speech-Language Pathology, 7*(3), 10–19.

Ingham, R. J., & Cordes, A. K. (1998b). On watching a discipline shoot itself in the foot. In N. Bernstein Ratner & E. C. Healy (Eds.), *Treat-*

ment and research: Bridging the gap. Hillsdale, NJ: Laurence Erlbaum Associates.

Onslow, M. (1992). Identification of early stuttering: Issues and suggested strategies. *American Journal of Speech-Language Pathology, 1,* 21–27.

Onslow, M. (1996). *Behavioral management of stuttering.* San Diego, CA: Singular Publishing Group.

Onslow, M. (1998, November). *Early stuttering: Nature's treatment, the Lidcombe Program, love, and the limits of science.* Paper read to the Annual Convention of the American Speech-Language-Hearing Association, San Antonio, TX.

Onslow, M., Andrews, C., & Lincoln, M. (1994). A control/experimental trial of an operant treatment for early stuttering. *Journal of Speech and Hearing Research, 37,* 1244–1259.

Onslow, M., Harrison, E., Jones, M., & Packman, A. (1998). Treating stuttering in young children: Predicting treatment time in the Lidcombe Program. *Journal of Speech, Language, and Hearing Research* (in review).

Packman, A., & Lincoln, M. (1998). Early stuttering and the Lidcombe Program: Deciding when to treat. *Advances in Speech Language Pathology* (in review).

Packman, A., & Onslow, M. (1998a). The behavioral data language of stuttering. In A. Cordes & R. J. Ingham (Eds.), *Treatment efficacy for stuttering: A search for empirical bases* (pp. 27–50). San Diego, CA: Singular Publishing Group.

Packman, A., & Onslow, M. (1998b). What is the take-home message from Curlee and Yairi? *American Journal of Speech-Language Pathology, 7*(3), 5–9.

Prins, D., & Ingham, R. J. (Eds.). (1983). *Treatment of stuttering in early childhood: Methods and issues.* San Diego, CA: College-Hill Press.

Rustin, L., & Cook, F. (1995). Parental involvement in the treatment of stuttering. *Language, Speech and Hearing Services in the Schools, 26,* 127–137.

Shenker, R. C., Kully, D., & Meltzer, A. (1998, August). Letter to the editor concerning the Leadership Conference. *Fluency and Fluency Disorders,* pp. 9–10.

Starkweather, C. W. (1997). Therapy for younger children. In R. F. Curlee & G. M. Siegel (Eds.), *Nature and treatment of stuttering: New directions* (2nd ed., pp. 257–279). Needham Heights, MA: Allyn & Bacon.

Watkins, R. V., & Yairi, E. (1997). Language production abilities of children whose stuttering persisted or recovered. *Journal of Speech, Language and Hearing Research, 40,* 385–399.

Yairi, E. (1997). Disfluency characteristics of childhood stuttering. In R. F. Curlee & G. M. Siegel (Eds.), *Nature and treatment of stuttering: New directions* (2nd ed., pp. 49–78). Needham Heights, MA: Allyn & Bacon.

Yairi, E., & Ambrose, N. (1992). A longitudinal study of stuttering in children: A preliminary report. *Journal of Speech and Hearing Research, 35,* 755–760.

Yairi, E., Ambrose, N., Paden, E. P., & Throneburg, R. N. (1996). Predictive factors of persistence and recovery: Pathways of childhood stuttering. *Journal of Communication Disorders, 29,* 51–77.

Zebrowski, P. M. (1997). Assisting young children who stutter and their families: Defining the role of the speech-language pathologist. *American Journal of Speech-Language Pathology, 6*(2), 19–28

Parent-Child Group Approach to Stuttering in Preschool Children

EDWARD G. CONTURE
KENNETH S. MELNICK

INTRODUCTION

This chapter describes the background, rationale, procedures, and typical outcome of a parent-child group approach to stuttering in preschool children. This approach was used for 17 years at Syracuse University and is now in the early stages of implementation at Vanderbilt University. Although it is difficult to fit this approach easily into the direct, indirect, or combined treatment categories discussed by Conture (1990) or Ramig and Bennett (1997), it is probably most appropriately considered an "indirect" approach. And it is fair to say that there is as much variety among different "indirect" methods as there is among different "direct" methods. For the time being, however, we will ignore such variation and try to focus on basic generalities among indirect approaches to the treatment of childhood stuttering.

To begin, Van Riper (1973) described indirect methods as those primarily focusing "on removing or reducing the stressful conditions presumably precipitating the disfluency . . . the therapists generally [seek] to keep the child from developing awareness of stuttering or fears of speaking so that the disorder will not progress . . . . efforts should be concentrated on altering parental attitudes, the family milieu and the conditions of communicative stress, with absolutely no interaction with the child himself" (p. 372). As we will try to show in this chapter, however, such a definition is a bit restrictive; that is, children can be and often are involved in modern-day indirect approaches. Indeed, children can learn to improve their speech fluency significantly by having appropriate adult models repeatedly presented to them. Likewise, as a result of indirect methods, children who stutter can learn simple communicative rules to follow when talking with peers and adults.

It is true that more than some of the children we initially evaluate (e.g., Yaruss, LaSalle, & Conture, 1998) will eventually recover with little or no intervention (e.g., Yairi & Ambrose, 1992; Yairi, Ambrose, & Niermann, 1993). It is just as true, as Kelly and Conture (1991) pointed out, that we presently have "no definite means for differentiating the child who will become a chronic stutterer from one encountering a temporary period of 'normal' even 'abnormal' disfluencies" (p. 309). In essence, we know that some children will recover on their own, we just don't know, in any absolute sense, whether the particular child we observe, at the time of initial evaluation, will be one of those who will or will not recover without treatment. Thus, we believe that it is incumbent upon us not to ignore a clinically significant problem (see Conture, 1997, p. 246, for further discussion of clinical significance). In other words, once we are reasonably clear that the problem will not "go away" on its own, we should actively, in as appropriate fashion as possible, attempt to treat the child and his or her problem.

While determining whether a child's stuttering will "go away" is far less than an exact science, some of the behaviors that we believe suggest that the child's stuttering is chronic and/or will not change without treatment include: (a) the child has been stuttering for 18 months or longer (Yairi, 1997); (b) more than 33% of the child's disfluency clusters are of the stuttering-stuttering variety (LaSalle & Conture, 1995); (c) the child scores 19 or higher on the Stuttering Severity Instrument for Children and Adults (Riley, 1994) and/or 17 or higher on the Stuttering Prediction Instrument for Young Children (Riley, 1981); (d) sound prolongations constitute 35% or more of the child's total stutterings (Yaruss, LaSalle, & Conture, 1998); this measure is the "sound prolongation index," employed by Schwartz and Conture (1988) to distinguish among subgroups of preschool children who stutter; and (e) eyeball movements to the side and/or eyelid blinking and the like occur during stuttering (Conture & Kelly, 1991). In our experience, the more of these behaviors exhibited by a preschool child, the stronger the risk that the child's problem is or will be chronic and will not remit without therapeutic intervention.

The above said, we should remember the adage that has guided generations of physicians: first of all, do no harm. Whatever intervention we initiate with the preschool child who stutters, we hope to do absolutely nothing to exacerbate or maintain the child's stuttering (as well as the family's inappropriate concerns about same) and hope to do many, many things to speed the child's recovery from stuttering. Keeping the preceding cautions in mind, we will now describe our parent-child group approach with preschool children.

In essence, as Kelly and Conture (1991) indicated, in our parent-child group, "we focus our attention on (a) providing children with 'tools' to assist them when they have difficulty communicating, and (b) providing their parents with information, suggestions, and opportunities for interacting with their child who stutters in a manner that facilitates fluency" (p. 309). Nothing, we repeat, nothing about this approach precludes subsequent use of more direct approaches, if that seems to be necessary. However, for most preschool children who stutter, we have found, as the first line of intervention, that these parent-child groups are very much in keeping with the adage "first of all, do no harm." That is, it is our experience that these groups do not exacerbate the child's stuttering. Quite to the contrary, in 70% or more of the preschool children we have treated with these groups, their stuttering significantly decreases to the point where the children are normally fluent or so minimally disfluent that important listeners (e.g., teachers, parents) do not notice or report noticing any speaking difficulties. Most importantly, we believe that, long after formal therapy has been discontinued, these parent-child groups provide the parents with the means to help maintain their child's recovery from stuttering.

Does this approach work with all children? Of course not. Does any approach? No treatment that we are aware of works for all people exhibiting the same problem. For example, some people are allergic to penicillin; some people suffer side effects from treatments so that the costs far outweigh the benefits; some people, through no fault of the health care provider, cannot or will not follow explicit, simple instructions and hence the treatment founders; and so forth. However, and as mentioned above, based on our experience of 17 years or more, we have found that our approach, for 70% of the children we treat, brings about a significant reduction in stuttering (resulting in an average stuttering frequency of 3% or less per 100 words of conversational speech).

Rationale

To draw an analogy, in the U.S.A., in the years immediately following World War II, when anti-Communist sentiments were at their strongest, it was said of the devoutly anti-Communist that they were so concerned about the "red peril," that they were looking for "reds under the bed." Well, almost to the same degree, some in our field have assumed that problems in the child's environment were the essential root cause of stuttering. Thus, these individuals diligently went looking for "environmental problems," and when they didn't find them, well, they found them anyway!

While both Wingate (1962) and Yairi (1997) appear to conclude that children who stutter have a greater chance than children who do not stutter of encountering unfavorable home conditions, Yairi (1997, p. 42) concurs with Adams (1993) that children who stutter, when taken as a group, are not raised in homes that can be considered "blatantly pathologic or palpably unhealthy emotionally" (a conclusion essentially the same as that of Schulze and Johannsen [1991] based on their review of relevant literature). As Adams noted, of course, it is still possible that "one or more major or subtle environmental variables not included in the studies reviewed may be operative" (p. 189).

For the time being, though, it is reasonable to assume that the environment of children who stutter is roughly within normal limits, or at least not "pathologic" or demonstrably "unhealthy emotionally." Why then bother with fixing something (i.e., the environment of children who stutter) that doesn't appear broken? Well, it is quite possible that environmental events do not have to be significantly broken (i.e., abnormal or pathological) to be a problem for a child. Besides, lest we forget, the child has a role in all of this. The child can, and often does, respond in less than fluency-facilitative ways to home environments that are overly but not pathologically or abnormally rushed, critical, competitive, interruptive, and the like.

Obviously, such child-specific behaviors are manifold and a thorough coverage of them goes well beyond the scope of the present chapter. However, we would like to discuss briefly the child's typical manner of responding to the environment and/or speaking difficulties/disfluencies to provide some balance to our previous discussion of the child's home environment. For example, Glasner (1949), based on his review of 70 case files of children who stutter, found that parents reported that their child's most common temperamental characteristic was "hypersensitivity." Although we lack a precise understanding of how, indeed whether, temperamental variables such as "hypersensitivity" influence childhood stuttering, recent years have witnessed increased interest in the role temperament plays in stuttering. For example, Felsenfeld (1997) recently suggested that "fast parental speech has deleterious consequence for fluency only for those children having a highly reactive temperament during a specific developmental period (e.g., 2 to 4 years)" (p. 18). Likewise, preliminary studies of Oyler (1996; Oyler & Ramig, 1995) indicated that children who stutter are significantly more behaviorally inhibited and temperamentally sensitive than children who do not stutter, according to parental responses to a paper-and-pencil scale, describing their child between 1 and 4 years of age. Oyler also has found preliminary evidence that children who stutter are significantly less likely to take risks than children who do not stutter, a finding consistent with Bloodstein's (1995) suggestion, based on his review of the literature, that "many stutterers are low . . . in willingness to risk failure" (p. 237). Clinically, Guitar (1997) recently provided an impressive number and variety of methods for treating children who stutter with apparently strong emotional responses to stuttering; responses that Guitar suggested may be related to some children's innate temperament. And while we try to deal routinely with such emotional responses in our parent-child groups, we agree with Guitar that these emotional responses to stuttering may be a large part of the reason some children are relatively resistant to treatment.

Therapeutically, within the context of our parent-child groups, we make some attempt to address the issues of emotionality and/or temperament through the parents. One of the primary ways we do this is by trying to help the parents adjust their physical, emotional, intellectual, and communicative environment in ways that accommodate their child's tendency to be (a) slow-to-warm-up to novel, different, or unfamiliar people, objects, and situations; (b) overly sensitive/reactive to environmental change, time pressures, anything strange or new, and the like; and (c) inappropriately fearful of objectively neutral environmental events, for example, loud noises, taking a bath, bugs, separation. Our experience suggests that such accommodations are often helpful in reducing some of the children's (a) frequent over-reaction to mistakes in their speech, (b) internal demands to be perfectly fluent, and (c) tendency not to attempt that which they feel they cannot do perfectly. The key, in all this, is not to attempt to rid the home environment of any and all variables that might negatively impact the child's speech fluency. Rather, the speech-language pathologist should attempt to provide parents with the "tools" needed to adjust the home environment at times when it appears things need to be neutralized and/or less problematic for the developing child.

Brief Overview of Pertinent Literature

Are we alone in believing that environmental changes are helpful for the child who stutters? Hardly. Johnson and his colleagues (1949, 1959) are well known for their advice to parents to be "good listeners, to understand the sequences of language and speech development, and not to be overly demanding of the child's linguistic skills" (1949, p. 154). Similarly Riley and Riley (1982) mentioned the importance of communicating with parents concerning any attitudes or behaviors possibly disruptive of their child's fluency. Bailey and Bailey (1982) have parents and significant others "monitor their respective speech and language patterns with reference to . . . rapidity, complexity and emotional intensity [advising the parents to] rush the child as infrequently as possible" (p. 29). Similarly, Rustin (1987) suggested that the family is "the main focus for early intervention with the young dysfluent child" and that family participation involves, among other factors, "parental training in the techniques of improving motor speech fluency" (p. 168).

More recently, Rustin, Botterill, and Kelman (1996) discussed various procedures to deal with parent-child interaction styles that may contribute to the child's stuttering, for example, parental reactions to disfluency, home routines, turn-taking, and the like. Ramig (1993) reasonably assumes that there are three interrelated levels (i.e., educational counseling, facilitating communication interaction, and parents as observers and participants) of parental involvement during treatment of childhood stuttering. Ramig and Bennett (1997) suggested that "clinicians need to incorporate environmental changes that facilitate fluency development into treatment plans" (p. 308). Manning (1996) suggested that research has demonstrated that "parents can be shown how to assist in altering the child's environment so that stuttering behavior is not maintained" (p. 115). In essence, more than a few workers in the field believe that parental involvement in treatment for childhood stuttering is not only desirable but crucial for therapeutic success.

Thus, there is nothing either novel or unorthodox about considering the impact of the environment on stuttering. Nearly

40 years ago, Johnson and Associates (1959) stated their well-known speculation that "the problem involves an interaction of at least two persons, a speaker and a listener. At the moment of onset of the problem the speaker is typically a child . . . and the listener is nearly always one of the child's parents, usually the mother" (p. 236). What appears to be a bit novel, in recent years, is the systematic consideration and implementation of changes dealing with the complex interaction between the child and the environment as it relates to stuttering. (For a recent, elegant attempt at making sense of the manifold possible interactions between the person who stutters, his or her innate abilities and his or her environment, see Smith & Kelly, 1997.) Specifically, in our parent-child groups, we focus, both individually and in combination, on the following three areas: (a) the young child who stutters, (b) the child's parents, and (c) the relationship between parent and child.

Parents: Why Involve Them?

Is it absolutely necessary to involve parents when treating children for stuttering? Of course not; speech-language pathologists frequently treat children who stutter with little or no parental involvement. For example, whether by design or due to circumstances, speech-language pathologists in the U.S.A., in both clinical as well as public school settings, often find themselves treating children who stutter with little or no involvement on the part of parents. And, we hasten to note, the converse occurs; clinicians sometimes "treat" only the parents. Indeed, parents-only intervention was fairly routine, at least for preschool and early elementary school-age children, during the time Johnson's (1955) diagnosogenic theory was preeminent. Furthermore, parents may be involved in the treatment of childhood stuttering in ways other than the classic procedures promulgated by strict adherents to the "indirect" approach to childhood stuttering (e.g., information sharing with parents, counseling or encouraging parents to use best parental practices in the raising of their child). Indeed, Onslow, Andrews, and Lincoln (1994) and Lincoln and Onslow (1997) recently reported an interesting, novel use of parents in the treatment of stuttering. In essence, following encouraging preliminary findings (Onslow et al., 1994), Lincoln and Onslow (1997), in a treatment study of 43 preschool children who stuttered, reported significant within-clinic reductions in stuttering through the use of a parent-conducted program of verbal response-contingent stimulation.

We contend, therefore, based on our clinical experience and knowledge of childhood stuttering, that the routine involvement of parents in the treatment of early childhood stuttering leads to better, more lasting improvement or recovery from stuttering. Logic dictates that we not isolate parents from appropriately assisting their child's speech and language development and improvement. We would not advocate such isolation any more than we would discourage parents' appropriate assistance of their child's academic, athletic, psychological, and social development and improvement. Even physicians, who often employ relatively "passive" treatments, for example, pills, injections, and so forth, must enlist the cooperation of parents to administer the treatments for children, to insure that the child gets adequate bed rest, fluids, food, reduced activities, and the like.

Particularly in the early stages of speech and language development, the child's parents often provide many of the spoken communication opportunities or "slots" that their child attempts to "fill" with his or her own spoken communication. With time, of course, as the content, form, and use of the child's spoken communication matures, the dynamic, bidirectional process of dialogic, spoken communication increasingly leads the child to generate or create opportunities or "slots" for their parents to "fill." Whatever the case, the foregoing discussion does not mean that we know, think, or are suggesting that parents cause stuttering. What it does mean, however, is that it is highly likely that parental behavior can impact the child's development to the good, bad, or indifferent.

Parental behavior has the real potential to exacerbate or maintain the child's stuttering and related behaviors; for example, Kelly and Conture (1992, Fig. 2, p. 1263) reported a strong, positive correlation ($\rho = 0.84$) between a child's stuttering severity and the duration of the mother-child "simultalk" (i.e., conversational overlaps between the child's and his or her mother's utterance). Again, this does not mean that parents cause their children to stutter; however, it does suggest that parental behavior is related, significantly so, to an existing stuttering problem. Indeed, as Conture and Zebrowski (1992) have said elsewhere, "If children and their behavior are immutable to the influences of their parents, why should we, as SLPs (speech-language pathologists), believe that these same children and their behavior are mutable to our therapeutic administrations?" (p. 127). If our behaviors as SLPs can influence a child, isn't it just as likely that the behaviors of a parent, who has much, much more contact with the child than we do, can and do influence the child's existing behavior? We think the answer is intuitive and logical, but we respect the right of others to disagree with us.

THE PROGRAM

Assessment

We have previously (Conture, 1990; Conture, 1997; Conture & Caruso, 1987; Conture & Yaruss, 1993) described, in considerable detail, our purpose, rationale for, and approach to the assessment of stuttering in children. Furthermore, there are other excellent sources regarding the evaluation of stuttering in children (Adams, 1977, 1980, 1991; Costello & Ingham, 1984; Culatta & Goldberg, 1995; Gregory & Hill, 1992; Hayhow, 1983; Ingham, 1985; Johnson, Darley, & Spriestersbach, 1963; Manning, 1996; Peters & Guitar, 1991; Pindzola, 1986; Pindzola & White, 1986; Rustin et al., 1996; Wall & Myers, 1995; Williams, 1974; Yaruss, 1997a; Zebrowski, 1994). In addition to these sources, it seems reasonable to suggest that recent advances in the measurement of stuttering (e.g., Cordes, Ingham, Frank, & Ingham, 1992; Howell, Sackin, & Glenn, 1997a, 1997b; Ingham, Cordes, & Finn, 1993) may some day lead to more reliable, valid measures of stuttering during routine diagnostic assessment. For example, the recent findings of Howell and colleagues (e.g., Howell et al., 1997b) suggested that we may eventually be able to use automatic recognition procedures (i.e., computer-assisted identification and classification) to locate and assess the stutterings of young children. Suffice it to say, given the amount of information available on assessment as well as advances in the measurement of stuttering, the future will witness continued improvements in the assessment and evaluation of childhood stuttering.

However, in a chapter focused on treatment, it seems sufficient to suggest that the assessment of childhood stuttering involves three general elements: (a) a case history form, filled out by the child's caregivers before or at the time of the evaluation; (b) an interview of the child's parents; and (c) a direct examination of the child. Based on a clinical sample of 100 children, our experience (Yaruss, LaSalle, & Conture, 1998) with preschool children who stutter at the time of initial evaluation suggested that about 10% of children will not require treatment, another 40% will require one or more re-evaluations before therapy is or is not recommended (with about 50%, or 20% of the total children initially evaluated, of those children re-evaluated being re-ferred for therapy), and 50% requiring immediate treatment of some form.

Explication of the exact behavior(s) associated with each of these diagnostic judgments goes well beyond the scope of this chapter; however, suffice it to say, for the present discussion, that the child's need for some form of intervention increases with the length of time since the onset of stuttering, the total number of disfluencies, the percent of the total disfluencies that are stut-tered, the greater percentage of sound prolongations per total stutterings, and the higher the scores on the Iowa Scale, the Stuttering Severity Instrument, and Stuttering Prediction Instru-ment. Whatever the nature and number of behaviors used to make diagnostic decisions, and regardless of what treatment procedure is eventually employed, it is reasonable to assume that therapy begins with a diagnostic evaluation.

It is a false economy to "save time" by doing a cursory as-sessment. As a television ad used to say, "it's pay me now or pay me later." A cursory, less than adequate assessment requires gaps to be filled during the first 4 to 8 weeks of therapy. The time saved by truncating the assessment is time spent during thera-py, trying to figure out the child's concerns, problems, needs, and the like rather than time spent treating the client. In our view, nothing is more important to successful treatment than successful assessment. The clinician should obtain sufficient breadth and depth of information to determine whether a prob-lem exists and the likelihood that it will continue, with or with-out treatment.

Equally, if not more important, is the opportunity assess-ment provides the clinician to orient the child and the child's family to the way in which the clinician views stuttering and plans for treatment to proceed. It would be unfortunate if the child and family begin treatment with very little understanding of the nature of the child's problem, what treatment will be about, and why. Indeed, information sharing with the parents, at the time of initial diagnosis as well as throughout treatment, is one very salient facet of "counseling" (Zebrowski & Schum, 1993).

One aspect of treatment—clinicians' understanding of and dealing with parental thoughts and feelings about the treatment process—begins at the time of initial diagnosis and continues throughout the treatment of children who stutter. For example, the clinician must help parents consider the consistency of their responses to their child, the consistency of their application of therapy strategies, the degree to which their child's behavior might be habituated, their expectations for rate and amount of change, the necessity of regular attendance of both parent and child, and so forth. It is not sufficient to merely open our clinical schedule and facilities to these children and their parents. Rather, the parents must, at the time of initial evaluation, be oriented to and understand what we are going to do, why we are going to do it, when, and how often.

At the end of the diagnostic, parents typically want to know three things: (a) Does my child stutter? (b) If the child does, will he or she outgrow it? and (c) If not, should therapy be initiated? Again, it is not the purpose of this chapter to delve into the details of assessment of childhood stuttering, the first author has done that elsewhere (e.g., Conture, 1997; Conture & Yaruss, 1993). Suffice it to say, if, after a thorough diagnostic, a child appears to be normally fluent, or at minimal or "no" risk for continuing to stutter, the child should probably be dismissed from further consideration. Such dismissal, however, does not preclude the speech-language pathologist, at the time of assessment or during subsequent phone calls, from spending some time counseling the parents and providing information to them about normal childhood development, both in general and specifically with regard to speech and language development. Conversely, these authors typically initiate therapy for children who, among other behaviors, have exhibited stuttering for 18 or more months, and whose stuttering appears to be frequently and regularly associated with physical tension, struggle, parental concern, and attendant with apparent frustration and/or fear. There is a "middle group," children whose total stuttering ranges from 3 to 7 per 100 words of conversational speech, who exhibit very little associated nonspeech behavior, and no apparent concern with, or awareness of, their stuttering or speech disfluencies. These children we typically view as being at "low" risk for continuing to stutter, and we evaluate them one or more additional times before therapy is initiated.

The Goal of Treatment

Although much of our diagnosis centers on the fluency of the child and things that help or hinder its development within the child, we should keep our eye on the prize: communication. The goal of therapy with children who stutter, we believe, is not merely achieving increased speech fluency but establishing the ability of the child to communicate whatever, wherever, whenever, and to whomever he or she wants. Communication, therefore, not fluency, is the ultimate goal of so-called "fluency" therapy.

We have made this same point elsewhere (Conture & Guitar, 1993) when discussing treatment efficacy with school-age children who stutter. In that context we stated that the goal of therapy should be to achieve speech that is functional in daily life activities, not speech that is 100% free from error, disfluency, and disruption. Similar notions have been put forth by Franken, van Bezooijen, and Boves (1997) about whether a client's speech fluency, as results from therapy, is "suitable" for various daily life activities. For example, what good would "improved fluency" be if (a) the child was reluctant to use these "improvements" in everyday life situations and/or (b) listeners felt this change in the child's speech was inappropriate for these situations, for example, answering questions, making requests, and meeting people. Speech-language pathologists have for too long paid too much attention, in our opinion, to the disability aspects of stuttering, that is, its behavioral manifestations, and far too little attention to the handicapping aspects of the disorder, that is, the academic, social, intellectual, vocational, and emotional disadvantages. Unfortunately, this trend is not likely to change any time soon, at least in the U.S. where third-party payments demand objective documentation of a client's problem, and change in that problem.

Our goals in the parent-child group are to help the child achieve, with parental facilitation and support, speech fluency that is functionally adequate to permit oral communication in daily life activities. Thus, with communication rather than totally fluent speech as the goal (the latter being something that few, if any, normally fluent speakers could achieve!), we are not concerned that some speech disfluencies remain, at the time of dismissal. Rather, our goal will be reached if the child and his/her parents demonstrate and feel that the child can communicate when and wherever he or she wants. In our opinion, the fact that a child achieves adequately fluent speech may be necessary but not sufficient for us to claim that our therapy was successful with that child. Instead, we believe, that the child needs to achieve communicatively adequate speech for us to have necessary as well as sufficient grounds for claiming therapeutic success. To draw an analogy, an individual may have a broken arm completely fixed (i.e., X rays indicate that it is completely mended), but be unable or unwilling to use it because of losing the habit of using the arm when it was in a cast and being fearful of rebreaking it or finding it weak after several weeks of disuse. Proof that an arm is mended is necessary but not sufficient to determine whether the person is or will be routinely using that arm for daily life activities.

The Treatment Program: Nature of Organization and Membership

In this section we describe the logistics of our program, the age range of the children in the program, and then the program itself.

Logistics

We have conducted our parent-child[1] groups in 12-week blocks of once-weekly, 45-minute therapy sessions in the mid to late afternoon. We have experimented with 6- to 8-week blocks to determine whether we can make decisions about (a) continuation of treatment, (b) discontinuation of treatment, and (c) changing the nature of treatment in a time frame shorter than 10 weeks. However, it appears that these decisions are more easily and efficiently made in 12-week rather than 6- to 8-week therapy blocks. Experience indicates that some children require 1 block of treatment, others 2 or 3, and a few 4 and more 12-week blocks of therapy before their fluency and related concerns (e.g., amount of apparent physical tension during stutterings, frustration with and/or fearfulness about talking) are sufficiently ameliorated to dismiss them from therapy. During these parent-child therapy sessions, the parents meet in a group (i.e., parent group) with a clinician, while the children meet in a separate group (i.e., child group). This separation of parent and child permits extensive adult-level discussion within the parent group and enhanced practice and interaction within the peer group. Parents also either observe part of their child's group and/or participate (near the end of the treatment session) in selected portions of the child's group to facilitate acquisition of fluency-enhancing skills by both children and parents for transfer to situations outside the clinic setting.

Age Range of Child Participants

Although this chapter focuses on children between 3 and 5 years old, it should be noted that we also conduct such groups for children 5–7, 8–10, and 11–13 years old. We group the children by age for purposes of number and nature of age-appropriate thera-

---

[1]The "parent-child group" has two aspects: a child group and a parent group, both of which meet in separate rooms but concurrently. To minimize the reader's confusion as much as possible, when we refer to the entire therapy program we use the phrase "parent-child group," when we refer to the child aspect of the parent-child group we use "child group," and when referring to the parent aspect of the parent-child group we use "parent group."

py activities, even though the underlying philosophy for groups remains the same: help the children learn how to change their stuttering and help their parents to support and foster the changes the children learn. Whatever age range clinicians use, they need to seriously consider grouping by age, for older children will act and state that they don't want to "play with babies" and younger children will act and state that they are intimidated, inhibited when interacting with "big kids." Usually the groupings that we have found to work are those stated above. Obviously, on the cusps between these age groupings, the clinician may be hard put to situate the child ideally in a group. Further, as any experienced clinician comes to realize, chronological age is not developmental age, and the wise clinician will consider both when selecting the group in which to place a child. For example, a 4.5-year-old who is developmentally advanced for his age might comfortably fit in a 5- to 7-year-old group.

From time to time, parents want to participate in the parent group without involving their child. We typically discourage this for several reasons, not the least being that the other parents feel it is inappropriate, unfair, or unwarranted for a set of parents to participate in the parent-child group without bringing their child. On the rare occasions when we have allowed parents to participate without their children, within 2 to 4 sessions, the parents almost invariably see the value of including their child, and begin to "lobby" us to "reconsider" and include their child in the child group. Conversely, we have some parents who initially agree to involve both their child and themselves in the group but for one reason or another find it less than desirable to interact with the other parents (e.g., a parent who finds that his or her standards for child-rearing are diametrically opposed to the bulk of the other parents).

The Program: Physical Arrangements

Ideally, the child group should involve two clinicians, one acting as group leader and the other assisting by demonstrating skills and activities, monitoring responses, and providing additional feedback, support, and reinforcement to the children. (However, one clinician can certainly perform both tasks.) It is especially helpful if the second clinician records each child's (dis)fluencies in real time, as the child speaks. We know from recent research (Yaruss, Max, Newman, & Campbell, 1998) that one can be reasonably confident, particularly during treatment, that on-line measurements of stuttering are sufficiently close to repeated off-line measurements of recordings.

We generally conduct the child group, for children 3–5 or 5–7 years old, on the floor, with each child being assigned a small rug. However, we also use age- or size-appropriate tables and chairs for certain activities, particularly activities with the parents during the last 10–15 minute session. In fact, to conduct effective treatment some form of "crowd control" is needed, in the form of fixed areas to sit. This is perhaps obvious, but it is difficult to either model for children fluency-enhancing activities or get them to practice these, if other children are roaming or running around the room. Some degree of control or order must be imposed to minimize and change unwanted behavior without inappropriately disrupting the ebb and flow of group dynamics. Providing each child with his or her own place to sit, on a chair or rug, helps a great deal in establishing the kind of gentle control needed for optimally effective therapy. Experienced clinicians will quickly recognize how something as simple as a piece of rug on the floor provides the structure needed for children who require such boundaries to adequately attend, cooperate and learn.

The Treatment Program: General Objectives

The parent-child stuttering group focuses on three areas, (a) communicative interactions, (b) speech production behaviors, and (c) attitudes about speech in general, especially parents' attitudes toward their own speech and that of their child. We suspect that point (b), modification of the child's speech production, will be adequately covered in other chapters in this book. Certainly, we have discussed this issue in considerable detail elsewhere (e.g., Conture, 1990, pp. 131–143) . "Easy speech," "hard speech," "smooth speech," "easy onsets," and the like should be familiar to the reader and if they are not there are many references describing these activities (see Ramig & Bennett, 1997, for a thorough coverage of their own direct treatment approaches with children as well as an excellent overview of various direct treatment procedures for children, e.g., Cooper & Cooper, 1985; Pindzola, 1987; Shine, 1980). While the majority of our child groups involve indirect approaches, when necessary, we employ direct procedures, especially for clients who seem to receive minimal benefit from the parent-child groups.

As we have mentioned elsewhere (Conture, 1990), most direct modifications of speech fluency involve, to some degree, changes in time (e.g., duration or length of articulatory contact) and tension (e.g., apparent or perceived level of muscle stiffness or contraction) of speech production. Although we believe it serves little purpose to label such procedures, because some may become more concerned with the label than the actual principle behind and procedure involved in the modification, our basic direct procedure would be most aptly described as an "easy movement forward." And although the following paragraph provides one example of our direct approach with preschool children, we believe it important to reiterate that a direct approach to stuttering with young children is not our typical first line of attack; rather, for us, direct treatment typically follows less than successful and/or protracted use of indirect therapy.

One example of our direct approach might involve the clinician trying to help the person who stutters change a fixed-articulatory contact (i.e., "block") on the word-initial /t/ in "time," a behavior typically associated with too much physical tension and inappropriately long articulatory contact. One means to change this behavior, by manipulating time and tension of speech production, involves the clinician requesting that the person who stutters "freezes" or holds the "block" even longer. While the child "holds onto the block," they gradually release the physical tension associated with the tongue-tip to alveolar ridge contact (for the /t/ sound) to the point where the person can move on, in this case, to articulate the vowel following the /t/. In essence, the clinician uses time-to-let-the-tension-go in attempts to help the client achieve speech that feels, looks, and sounds more fluent. After the child is taught and demonstrates an understanding of this procedure, the clinician can ask the child to make the stutterings "easier," to "move out" of them with less physical tension. Again, to achieve this gradual release in physical tension, the child is instructed to use more time; that is, there is an increase in time to achieve a decrease in tension. To help the child understand and achieve this procedure, we use the analogy of a tightly clenched fist that is opened slowly to gradually release physical tension (see Guitar's therapy demonstration in Conture, Guitar, & Fraser, 1997); while practicing this analogy, the child may, for example, hold the articulatory posture for the word-initial /p/ in "pop" longer, but in so doing gradually release the tension so that he or she can move on to the posture for the subsequent vowel.

However, rather than dwelling on direct approaches to stuttering in preschool children, which constitute a minority rather than a majority of our efforts with these children, we would rather focus on (a) communicative interactions between the child and parent, (b) parental attitudes about speech in general, their own speech and that of their child, and how (a) is influenced by (b) and vice versa.

Communicative Interactions

We attempt to steer child groups and parent groups toward common ground. In the *child* group, the child is taught (through modeling and direct instruction) the following rules of communicative interaction:

- Listen (when someone else is talking)
- Wait (your turn to talk)
- Don't talk (when someone else is talking).

In the *parent* group, the parents are taught (through modeling and direction instruction) that the following parental communicative behaviors and interactions do not facilitate the child's speech fluency:

- Frequent interruptions of their child, or talking as their child talks (i.e., "simultalk," see Conture & Caruso, 1987, p. 101)
- Talking for their child
- Frequent use of long, complex utterances even when discussing simple matters, answering simple questions, or making simple requests
- Excessively rapid rates of utterance
- Frequent corrections of each and every speech "mistake" the child makes.

Early in the treatment program, we ask the child's parents to observe their own speech behaviors (paying particular attention to the bulleted points above) during interactions with their children as well as with each other in their child's presence. We ask the parents to be prepared to discuss and analyze these behaviors at subsequent parent group meetings. When the parents seem ready and willing to change these behaviors, we request that they do so during daily activities (5 to 10 minutes per activity) with their child, for example, at the breakfast table, at the dinner table, when reading a story at bedtime, while driving in the car, and so forth.

We typically start by having the parents delay about 1 second before responding to their child, to minimize the frequency and duration of their interruptions of their child (such interruptions typically occurring during the mid to latter part of their child's utterances). Indeed, in our opinion, if the parent cannot or will not minimize his or her interrupting, talking for, or talking over the child, it will be difficult for any treatment to work, indirect or direct. These behaviors encourage the child to speed up both the planning for as well execution of his or her utterances, neither of which is a fluency-facilitating behavior. To ensure that the parents do this every day, we encourage them to select one activity and stick to making changes in their speech during that activity each day rather than switching among activities each day. We emphasize to the parents that they should monitor and modify their own speech, rather than the speaking behavior of the other parent. Otherwise, if the mother begins to focus on the father's behavior and vice versa, it can become a source of marital friction and we don't want to engender that, if we can at all avoid it.

Again, we are not suggesting that the aforementioned parental behaviors (e.g., frequent interruptions of the child's utterances) cause stuttering, only that their habitual presence appears to exacerbate and/or maintain a child's disfluent speech behavior. Most children in the group become quite fluent rather quickly with a clinician who is using very slow, physically relaxed speech. Of course, this is not the same as the home or even a more communicatively pressured clinical situation (see Yaruss, 1997b, for data describing how stuttering changes across different speaking situations). Nor is it supposed to be. This "slower, easier" style of communication is purposeful, it is used by the clinicians to help the children become as fluent as possible (and again, we remind the reader that, for most children, no direct treatment of their speech will be required). Why as fluent as possible? First and foremost, we want to help the children to experience more fluent speech, to be better able to communicate more freely when they want, about what they want, to whom they want. Another important reason is that we want the parents to see that (a) their children can be more fluent, and (b) if they attempt to make the changes in parental communicative behaviors and interactions that we suggest, their child's speech fluency can be improved.

Usually, at this point, parents ask, "Am I going to have to talk that slowly *all* the time?" To this we answer: Absolutely not. We are modeling for the child a rather pronounced, but not unnaturally so, slow, physically relaxed speaking behavior in the child's group. The parents see this, see that it works, but worry that (a) they won't be able to do it or (b) they won't be able to do it all the time. We assure them that the model is exaggerated to help them recognize the changes that they will make. We also assure them that we want them to "move" from their often rapid, interrupting, and long, complex utterances to more normal rates, levels of interruption, and complexity. It is not unusual for parents, with all good intentions, to talk for and/or interrupt their child to "help" the child deal with his or her stuttering. And indeed, as most SLPs who work with the parents of children who stutter will attest, the vast majority of parental behaviors are driven by love, concern, and an intense desire to help their child whom they perceive as frustrated, worried, and fearful.

In our experience, parental intentions are typically noble. Where these writers take exception, at least with some parents, is with certain parental methods to "improve" their child's oral communication. We hasten to point out, however, that stuttering is not the only problem where sincere, caring individuals have engaged in nonproductive procedures or procedures that actually exacerbated the very problem they were meant to improve! For example, concerned citizens and/or government agencies have imported birds, animals, and insects to treat one problem, only to have the imported bird, animal, or insect become a problem in its own right. Our point? Merely this: Poor procedures can stem from the purest and most sincere of purposes.

With stuttering, for example, well-meaning, caring caregivers as well as other adults can imbue in their child, through instruction and example, the belief that mistakes in one's speech are to be ashamed of, avoided, corrected, or hidden. For example, we recently evaluated a 3-year, 10-month-old boy whose instances of stuttering (about 10% during conversational speech) were often associated with physical tension, pitch rises, and inappropriate nonspeech behaviors. This boy told us several times during our routine assessment of his phonology and expressive language, that the examining speech-language pathologist "didn't talk right," that she "said that sound wrong"! Such critical attitudes on the part of children, in our experience, are almost invariably learned, that is, through adult model, instruction, or correction. On questioning, we learned that the father was teaching the child Spanish (as a second language) and a good

deal of attention was paid to the pronunciation of sounds, syllables, and words, with frequent review and reiteration of "inappropriate" pronunciation. (It should be noted that this child, in
English phonology, exhibited 10 phonological processes; thus,
his ability to quickly, sequentially, and accurately produce the
sounds of his native language was less than well developed.) Did
such "drill and correction" on the part of the father lead this
child to be overly critical of the accuracy of speech production?
We, of course, do not know that for a fact, but it was most curi-
ous that the child frequently mentioned the accuracy of our
speech and routinely exhibited physically tense attempts to correct his own less than adequate speech productions.

What are we trying to say? Just this: We try very, very hard
not to question the sincerity, caring, concern, or intentions of the
parent. We try to support the parents fully in their love and concern for their child, all the while concentrating on helping them
develop behaviors, methods, and procedures that help rather
than hinder the development of the child's fluency. We reiterate
to the parents that if producing these behaviors (e.g., minimizing
the frequency and duration of the time they spend talking while
their child is talking) was easy they wouldn't need us. Likewise,
we tell them that if what they were doing to "improve" their
child's speech and language behavior actually worked, they
wouldn't be attending our clinic! Parents generally get the point.
If what they are or were doing, regardless of how pure their intentions, was effective, they would not have needed to seek help.
This quickly, in our experience, helps them "get with the program" and explore alternative methods. After all, what do they
have to lose? What they are or were doing certainly isn't working.

Among the many things parents can learn to do that really
seem to help their child, (a) reduction of talking while their child
is talking and (b) waiting about 1 second before responding to
their child seem most effective. Time and again, parents tell us
that these two behaviors, although at first difficult and somewhat artificial, seem to help their child's fluency. Why? We, of
course, don't know for certain. However, it is our hypothesis that
reduction of "simultalking" and increase in the turn-switching
pause or parental response time latency helps the child:

- ■ Spend more time planning his or her utterances; that
  is, the child may take more time to plan the utterance
  because he feels that mom or dad is less apt to interrupt or finish his sentence.

- Speak at a more appropriate rate; that is, the child may take more time to produce the utterance, feeling that mom or dad is less apt to complete the utterance or interrupt.
- Process (or concentrate on processing) his or her own utterance rather than having to simultaneously monitor and/or process that as well as the parent's utterance.

Some basic questions with this change, as with all changes in parental behavior, are: when, where, and how often? Frequently parents, in a sincere but often overly enthusiastic attempt to help, try to make the change every time they talk with the child. This is neither possible nor necessary. As we stated before, in the beginning, parents should be given 1 to 3 times or places per day when they can practice the change with their child, such as during the morning or evening ritual, when in the car, at the dinner table, or when reading to the child. We would far rather the parents "pause a second before responding" in one 5-minute conversation every day than in one 60-minute conversation once a week! What we are striving for is the parents' eventual ability to use this or any change in communicative interaction at any time they feel they need to rather than during every single waking minute of conversation with the child. We do not want to shackle the parents to a modification ball-and-chain they must drag around and through each and every conversation they have with the child. That is not only unnecessary but counterproductive in the long run. For if the parents sense or feel that they must always engage in X, Y, or Z interaction, even when their child is reasonably fluent, they will eventually stop doing it because of the sheer amount of effort, energy, and time it takes. Simply put, the parents will give up. Rather, we want them to realize that the change in behavior should become second-nature to them, to use when the child is having difficulties or showing a tendency to backslide into older, less facilitative behavior.

Speech Production Behavior

In our earlier discussions of our parent-child group and related therapy approaches (e.g., Conture, 1990; Kelly & Conture, 1991), we described in some detail means by which we might change the speech production behavior of preschool and early elementary school-aged children who stutter. Since those publications, we have moved somewhat away from this earlier position, at least during a child's initial parent-child group. Why? We have increasingly found that the changes in communication interactions detailed above, for both child and parent, have been necessary as well as sufficient in many cases. After 12 to 24 sessions, however, it may become apparent that, for some children, such changes are not sufficient to bring about meaningful and/or long-term change. These children generally need more individual attention and/or direct approaches. However, it is our experience that, even with these children, the eventual use of more direct procedures is facilitated by demonstrating as well as discussing in the child's group the concepts of physical tension and relaxation in speech and related activities, for example, writing with a tense versus a more relaxed grip.

To do this, we borrow from Williams' (1971) dichotomous concept of "hard" versus "easy" speech. This concept describes, at a cognitive-linguistic level most children can understand, the complex interactions between time and physical tension that are at the heart of disfluent speech production. Children are helped to recognize and produce different types of "easy" as well as "hard" speech. Using these concrete, less abstract labels seems to have meaning for the children. In essence, by employing more concrete, everyday terminology, we believe it is a bit easier for the child to grasp the idea behind as well as actual mechanics of the behaviors we want them to perform and/or change.

As described in Kelly and Conture (1991), we use terms like "big bumps" for whole-word repetitions, "little bumps" for sound/syllable repetitions, "skidding" for sound prolongations, and "getting stuck" for blocks. The emphasis here is not on generation of clever terms but on what children who stutter are physically doing and feeling when they stutter and how that may differ from when they do not stutter. The terms we use are a means not an end to get the children quickly and easily to feel and change what they are doing, to "make speech easier." The clinician—and this is very important—should be able and willing to demonstrate, model, and show the child what to do; how to make, for example, "getting stuck" sound, look, and feel easier (i.e., shorter and less physically tense). We are interested here in a "stutter more easily" rather than a "speak more fluently" approach. In our opinion, proactive procedures, for example, parental behaviors that indirectly encourage the child to take more time to plan and execute utterances, are important, for both the parent and child. However, for some children, reactive strategies that involve directly modifying the child's speech behavior, for example, "make that easier," are also needed.

In other words, regardless of what treatment a child has experienced, from time to time, children will experience certain sounds, syllables, words, situations, listeners, and so forth where they have difficulty talking fluently and will exhibit "hard" speech. Instead of trying to expunge all such difficulties or disfluencies, instead of having, in effect, zero tolerance for stuttering, we believe it far more appropriate to prepare our young clients for how to handle the occasional stuttering. Our strategy here is "reactive" in that we try to have the children learn to recognize and appropriately react to an instance of stuttering, despite the fact that both they and their parents have been proactively attempting to facilitate fluency.

Let us reiterate that we do not usually begin our parent-child groups with direct attempts to modify the child's stuttering. When we do engage in direct approaches, for example, with a child for whom an indirect approach was minimally successful, we want to ensure that whatever means we use to bring out such change—stutter more easily, speak more fluently or some combination of the two—leads to fluent speech that sounds natural[2] and, ideally, suitable (see Franken et al., 1997) for most speaking situations. Clinicians should be aware of the fact that communication, not fluency, is the ultimate goal of treatment. Of what value would it be, to draw an analogy, to set and mend a person's broken leg so that the person could or would not use it? Likewise, of what value would it be to provide someone with fluent, but unnatural speech that he or she wouldn't use for communication? Providing the child and his or her parents with strategies that are functional, natural, and suitable for all normal communication purposes should be our goal, rather than imbuing the child, the child's parents, and ourselves with zero tolerance for errors, mistakes, or disfluencies in everyday conversational speech.

EVALUATION

At the time of this writing we have treated over 200 preschool children in our parent-child groups. We determine that a child is ready for dismissal when he or she exhibits adequate but not to-

---

[2]See Manning (1996, pp. 222–228) for a good overview of this topic. We are not suggesting that clinicians must always apply, for example, Martin, Haroldson, and Triden's (1984) 9-point scale for rating speech naturalness of the posttreatment speech of children who stutter (something that has rarely been documented in a report of treatment published in a peer-reviewed scholarly journal).

tal fluency, that is, an average of 3% or less stutterings per 100 words across an 8-week period. Our records indicate that 70% of our young clients become "ready for dismissal" 12 to 36 weeks from the time of treatment onset. While perhaps obvious, being ready for dismissal is not the same as being dismissed. That is, being "ready for dismissal" signals a period of time where the child and parents can change from once-per-week to once-every-other-week treatment, the beginning of the transfer phase, which is discussed later. Typically, being ready for dismissal takes two 12-week "blocks" of consecutive treatment, with some obtaining this in one 12-week block and others needing as many as four or more 12-week blocks. Success, we hasten to point out, is a relative not an absolute term. Figure 2–1 shows the stuttering frequency data exhibited by one such "successful" case. Note that we report not just stuttering frequency but the frequency of all disfluencies (including phrase repetitions). At the risk of putting too fine a point on the matter, we do ourselves and the parents of the preschool child a disservice when we imply or make explicit that our treatment will result in zero disfluency. Zero disfluency is an impossibility, because the speech of normally fluent children (teenagers and adults) contains some speech disfluencies; just very few, if any, stutterings. In other words, does it

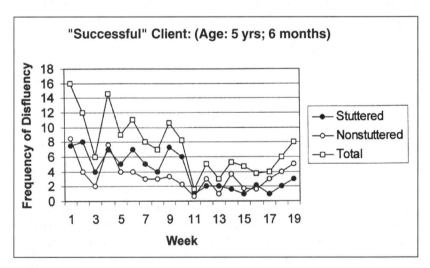

Figure 2–1. A "successful" client. Percentages of stuttered, nonstuttered, and total (stuttered + nonstuttered) disfluencies for the first 19 weeks of therapy. For this client, both stuttered (i.e., sound syllable repetitions, whole-word repetitions, and prolongations) and total disfluencies have decreased (i.e., the child's stuttering appears to be improving). Nonstuttered disfluencies (i.e., multisyllabic whole-word repetitions, interjections, phrase repetitions, and revisions) have remained relatively consistent.

make sense to make the speech of children who stutter more fluent than that of children who do not stutter? We don't think so. Figure 2–2 shows the stuttering frequency data exhibited by a more "volatile" case. This child's stuttering was quite variable, requiring more and/or different forms of treatment. Children represented by Figure 2–2, we estimate, represent 25–30% of our total patient population, with about 50% going on, eventually, to be successful and the other 50% being nonsuccessful, requiring different forms of treatment. Figure 2–3 shows stuttering frequency data exhibited by a nonchanging or "nonsuccessful" client. This child, after some initial changes, showed little or no change for several weeks. Children such as those represented by Figure 2–3 typically require different forms and/or schedules of therapy. Such "unsuccessful" clients exist regardless of approach, and their presence needs to be taken into consideration. Some of these children eventually stabilize and become adequately fluent; others require discontinuation of treatment, change in treatment, or referral elsewhere.

As an aside, we would like to mention the fact that we have always assessed and considered what percentage of the total disfluencies are stuttered. We have used this measure to help us

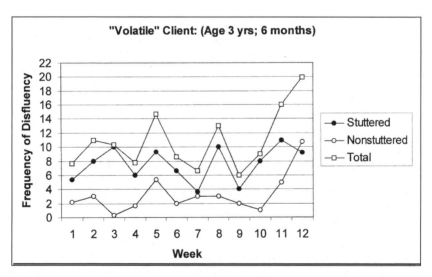

Figure 2–2. A "volatile" client. Percentages of stuttered, nonstuttered, and total (stuttered + nonstuttered) disfluencies for the first 12 weeks of therapy. For this client, both stuttered (i.e., sound syllable repetitions, whole-word repetitions, and prolongations) and total disfluencies have varied tremendously (i.e., the child's stuttering appears to be quite volatile). Nonstuttered disfluencies (i.e., multisyllabic whole-word repetitions, interjections, phrase repetitions, and revisions) have also varied.

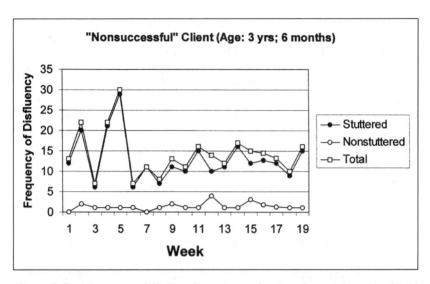

Figure 2–3. A "nonsuccessful" client. Percentages of stuttered, nonstuttered, and total (stuttered + nonstuttered) disfluencies for the first 19 weeks of therapy. For this client, stuttered (i.e., sound syllable repetitions, whole-word repetitions, and prolongations) and total disfluencies have varied considerably initially, but appear to be essentially nonchanging. Likewise, little or no change in nonstuttered disfluencies (i.e., multisyllabic whole-word repetitions, interjections, phrase repetitions, and revisions) is apparent.

classify children as stutterers as well as to monitor the child's progress in treatment. For example, if a child exhibits on average a total of 10 disfluencies per 100 words and of these 5 are stuttered, we would say the child exhibits 50% stutterings per total disfluencies. And if, after a period of treatment, this value for this child dropped from 50% to 30%, we would report that the child is making progress (making progress, of course, is not the same as success, but is movement in the right direction). Recently, our use of the "percent stutterings per total disfluencies" has been reinforced by Yairi's (1997) observation that, on the average, across eight studies of children who stutter, 72% of the total disfluencies were stutterlike, a percentage two to three times that of children who do not stutter (i.e., 25–40%). If as a result of treatment, the percent stutterings per total disfluencies, regardless of the absolute total number of disfluencies, approaches 25–40%, we believe one can meaningfully consider the child to be approaching the point of being "disfluent within normal limits."

The key question, of course, is whether "successful" clients maintain their changes over time (i.e., whether there is adequate transfer or carryover). Obviously, there is no one-size-fits-all solution to the important problem of transfer. And, after all, the goal of treatment is not change in the clinic, but change outside the clinic. The goal is to help the child to be able to communicate freely in the "real-world," during everyday, routine daily activities, not only during therapy sessions. In the beginning, to try to assess whether we had met our treatment goals, we would follow up our clients every 6–18 months for 5 years after dismissal; in recent years we have discontinued that practice. Instead, we have dealt with issues pertaining to maintenance in two related ways: (a) building maintenance into treatment, and (b) letting the parents "dictate" dismissal.

First, we attempt to assess maintenance by monitoring the child's progress as he or she moves from once-a-week to once-every-other week sessions. We call this "phasing out of treatment," and it is something "built into" the treatment plan and an aspect of our program described to parents from the beginning. If the child maintains fluency, we shift to once-per-month sessions, and if the child maintains fluency at that frequency of treatment we shift to once every other month. From once every other month, we shift to once every 3 months and then once every 6 months. Typically, sometime in the once every 3 months to once every 6 months, the parents ask to be dismissed. However, we try to maintain the client through the twice a year (once every 6 months) phase. Very few, if any clients, challenge our decision to dismiss their child once the child is maintaining adequate fluency when seen twice per year.

Second, we try to let parents "dictate" dismissal. We have found, through long experience, that our objective criteria for dismissal are not as important as parental feelings that the child has improved. In essence, we tell the parent that the child is, in our opinion, ready for dismissal, but we actively solicit the parent's opinion. If the parent is uncertain—implicitly or explicitly indicating lack of readiness to cut the clinical umbilical cord—we defer to the parent's request . For example, recently we felt a 4-year-old girl was ready for once-a-month treatment but the parents felt otherwise, given the impending arrival of a new baby. The parents felt that they needed the twice per month schedule to continue during the first month or so of adjustment and excitement in the home with the new baby. We agreed to their request. In essence, our experience indicates that the child will quickly return to our clinic with a "relapse" problem, if the parents are not ready for the child to be dismissed. Thus, by allowing parents to decouple from treatment at their own rate, we have found that far fewer of our clients return for treatment. Naturally, during the time when we believe the child to be ready but the parents do not, we continually talk with and support the parents in their decision and observation. We find it helps during this period to point out to the parent the child's progress, how the child is handling formerly difficult situations, how the child's behavior is so much improved. Using charts such as those depicted in Figures 2–1 through 2–3 helps immensely, and we recommend their use to clinicians for both data gathering and description as well as for parent information-sharing.

As noted, approximately 30% of our young clients do not meet, within a reasonable time frame, our criteria for being ready for dismissal. Although many variables obviously account for such difficulties, the following are a few of the "red flags" we have noted: (a) poor attendance (a universal sign, we assume); (b) parents who cannot or will not fully participate in the parent part of the group; (c) children whose temperament is that of the "slow-to-warm-up" or "behaviorally inhibited" child, for example, a child with strong fears, who is overly reactive to environmental change, minimizes contact with other children, and has persistent, marked difficulties separating from the parent; (d) children with concomitant speech and language problems; (e) children and/or parents where emotional discomfort and/or anxiety is so pervasive as to require individual and/or family counseling; and (f) children with attention deficit disorders.

A percentage of our less than successful clients become successful over time. We call these "protracted" cases; if these "protracted" cases were added to our original 70% we would report a success rate of approximately 80% of our young clients. A percentage of the remaining 20% may get adequately fluent, but not in the context and/or as a result of our parent-child group.

SUMMARY

- The purpose of this chapter was to describe the background, rationale, purpose, procedures, and evaluation of a parent-child stuttering group. It was suggested, in the background section, that stuttering involves a complex interaction between the child's environment and the innate abilities the child brings to that environment. Thus, in our opinion, parental involvement in treatment for childhood stuttering is not only desirable but crucial for therapeutic success. This does not mean that we know, think, or suggest that parents cause stuttering. What it does mean, however, is that it is highly likely that parental behavior can impact the development of the child.

■ The rationale for this indirect approach is that by "reducing the stressful conditions presumably precipitating the disfluency the child (can be kept) from developing awareness of stuttering or fears of speaking so that the disorder will not progress. . . . this can be done by altering parental attitudes, the family milieu and the conditions of communicative stress." It is believed that the clinician should repeatedly employ appropriate adult models when communicating with the child, as well as having the child learn simple communicative rules to follow when talking with peers. The parent-child groups discussed in this chapter focus, both individually and in combination, on the following three areas: (a) the young child who stutters, (b) the child's parents, and (c) the special relationship between parent and child because of the child's stuttering.

■ While the parents are meeting in one room, the children meet in another. Near the end of the session, the parents are brought together with the children for a planned parent-child activity. The general objectives of the children's group are modification of (a) communicative interactions, (b) speech production behaviors, and (c) attitudes about speech in general, the children's speech in particular, and themselves as speakers.

■ Clinicians and parents show rather than tell the child what to do. Whether the clinician is trying to help the child deal with communicative stress, learn more fluency-appropriate means of speaking, or change stutterings from long, physically tense to short, physically more relaxed, the emphasis is on the clinician modeling the behavior desired. The objectives for the parent group, to help them better understand and change their own and their children's communicative interactions and behaviors, are brought about through (a) counseling and information sharing, (b) guided observations of the children interacting with the clinician, and (c) guided participation in therapy with the children and clinicians.

■ To date, it appears that 70% of the children who participate in these groups are "ready for dismissal" (8 weeks or more exhibiting 3% or less stuttering per 100 words in conversational speech) as a result of treatment. Most children take one to two 12-week blocks of treatment to reach this point; some do so in one block, others require three to five blocks. Approximately one third of the 30% who fail require protracted treatment before success is achieved. Experience indicates that it is important that therapy be gradually curtailed, changing from once a week to every other week to once a month to every other month, to twice a year to once a year. This gradual phase-out procedure has led to a less than 10% relapse rate.

- The approach eschews a one-size-fits-all treatment plan; instead we try to let the quantity and quality of the child's treatment plan be dictated by the child's behavior and progress, the parent's behavior and progress, and the interactions between parents and child. Although between 20 to 30% of the children who enter these groups may eventually require "direct" treatment for stuttering and/or referral to other professionals, for the typical child these groups bring about appreciable change within about 4 to 6 months, and over the next 6 to 18 months of phase-out treatment these changes stabilize and generalize to a greater number and variety of speaking situations. However, the parents are told from the beginning not to expect total (for all normal purposes) fluency, that the goal for the parent-child group is functionally adequate speech. The emphasis is on communication. We strive to help the child talk about what he or she wants to talk about, when, where, and to whomever he or she wants.

Acknowledgment

Preparation of this manuscript was supported in part by an NIH grant (DC00523) to Vanderbilt University. Development and conduct of our parent-child groups have been made possible through the assistance of the following dedicated colleagues: Amy Egnew, Susan Finkenstadt, Jennifer Ask, Ellen Kelly, Christine Laney, Lisa LaSalle, Kenneth Logan, Linda Louko, Lesley Wolk, Scott Yaruss, and Patricia Zebrowski. Special thanks to the many children and their parents we have had the privilege to know, and from whom we have learned so much about stuttering, the therapy process, and ourselves.

REFERENCES

Adams, M. (1977). A clinical strategy for differentiating the normally nonfluent child and the incipient stutterer. *Journal of Fluency Disorders, 2*, 141–148.

Adams, M. (1980). The young stutterer: Diagnosis, treatment, and assessment of progress. *Seminars in Speech, Language, and Hearing, 1*, 289–299.

Adams, M. (1991). The assessment and treatment of the school-age stutterer. *Seminars in Speech and Language, 12*, 279–290.

Adams, M. (1993). The home environment of children who stutter. *Seminars in Speech and Language, 14*, 185–189.

Bailey, A., & Bailey, W. (1982). Managing the environment of the stutterer. *Journal of Communication Disorders, 6*, 26–39.

Bloodstein, O. (1995). *A handbook on stuttering* (5th ed.). San Diego, CA: Singular Publishing Group, Inc.

Conture, E. G. (1990). *Stuttering* (2nd ed.). Englewood Cliffs, NJ: Prentice-Hall.

Conture, E. G. (1997). Evaluating childhood stuttering. In R. F. Curlee & G. M. Siegel (Eds.), *Nature and treatment of stuttering* (2nd ed., pp. 239–256). Needham Heights, MA: Allyn & Bacon.

Conture, E., & Caruso, A. (1987). Assessment and diagnosis of childhood disfluency. In L. Rustin, D. Rowley, & H. Purser (Eds.), *Progress in the treatment of fluency disorders* (pp. 84–104). London: Taylor & Francis.

Conture, E., & Guitar, B. (1993). Evaluating efficacy of treatment of stuttering: School-age children. *Journal of Fluency Disorders, 18*, 253–287.

Conture, E., Guitar, B., & Fraser, J. (1997). Therapy in action: The school-age child who stutters [Videotape]. Memphis, TN: Stuttering Foundation of America.

Conture, E., & Kelly, E. (1991). Young stutterers' nonspeech behaviors during stuttering. *Journal of Speech and Hearing Research, 34*, 1041–1056.

Conture, E. G., & Yaruss, J. S. (1993). *Handbook for childhood stuttering: A training manual.* Tucson, AZ: Bahill Intelligent Computer Systems.

Conture, E. G., & Zebrowski, P. (1992). Can childhood speech disfluencies be mutable to the influences of speech-language pathologists, but immutable to the influences of parents? *Journal of Fluency Disorders, 17*, 121–130.

Cooper, E., & Cooper, C. (1985). *Personalized fluency control therapy.* Allen, TX: DLM.

Cordes, A., Ingham, R., Frank, P., & Ingham, J. (1992). Time-interval analysis of interjudge and intrajudge agreement for stuttering event judgements. *Journal of Speech and Hearing Research, 35*, 483–494.

Costello, J. M., & Ingham, R. J. (1984). Assessment strategies for stuttering. In R. F. Curlee & W. H. Perkins (Eds.), *Nature and treatment of stuttering: New directions* (pp. 303–333). San Diego, CA: College-Hill Press.

Culatta, R., & Goldberg, S. (1995). *Stuttering therapy: An integrated approach to theory and practice.* Boston: Allyn & Bacon.

Felsenfeld, S. (1997). Epidemiology and genetics of stuttering. In R. F. Curlee & G. M. Siegel (Eds.), *Nature and treatment of stuttering* (2nd ed., pp. 3–23). Needham Heights, MA: Allyn & Bacon.

Franken, M. C., van Bezooijen, R., & Boves, L. (1997). Stuttering and communicative suitability of speech. *Journal of Speech, Language, and Hearing Research, 40,* 83–94.

Glasner, P. (1949). Personality characteristics and emotional problems in stutterers under the age of five. *Journal of Speech and Hearing Disorders, 14,* 135–138.

Gregory, H. H., & Hill, D. (1992). Differential evaluation, differential therapy for stuttering children. In R. F. Curlee (Ed.), *Stuttering and related disorders of fluency* (pp. 23–44). New York: Thieme Medical Publishers.

Guitar, B. (1997). Therapy for children's stuttering and emotions. In R. F. Curlee & G. M. Siegel (Eds.), *Nature and treatment of stuttering* (2nd ed., pp. 280–291). Needham Heights, MA: Allyn & Bacon.

Hayhow, R. (1983). The assessment of stuttering and the evaluation of treatment. In P. Dalton (Ed.), *Approaches to the treatment of stuttering.* London: Croom Helm.

Howell, P., Sackin, S., & Glenn, K. (1997a). Development of a two-stage procedure for the automatic recognition of dysfluencies in the speech of children who stutter: I. Psychometric procedures appropriate for selection of training material for lexical dysfluency classifiers. *Journal of Speech, Language, and Hearing Research, 40,* 1073–1084.

Howell, P., Sackin, S., & Glenn, K. (1997b). Development of a two-stage procedure for the automatic recognition of dysfluencies in the speech of children who stutter: II. ANN recognition of repetitions and prolongations with supplied word segment markers. *Journal of Speech, Language, and Hearing Research, 40,* 1085–1096.

Ingham, R. J. (1985). Assessment of stuttering in children. In J. Gruss (Ed.), *Stuttering therapy: Prevention and early intervention.* Memphis, TN: Speech Foundation of America.

Ingham, R., Cordes, A., & Finn, P. (1993). Time-interval measurement of stuttering: Systematic replication of Ingham, Cordes, and Gow (1993). *Journal of Speech and Hearing Research, 32,* 1168–1176.

Johnson, W. (1949). An open letter to the mother of a stuttering child. *Journal of Speech Disorders, 14,* 3–8.

Johnson, W. (1955). The time, the place, and the problem. In W. Johnson (Ed.), *Stuttering in children and adults.* Minneapolis, MN: University of Minnesota Press.

Johnson, W., & Associates. (1959). *The onset of stuttering: Research findings and implications.* Minneapolis, MN: University of Minnesota Press.

Johnson, W., Darley, F., & Spriestersbach, D. (1963). *Diagnostic methods in speech pathology.* New York: Harper.

Kelly, E. M., & Conture, E. G. (1991). Intervention with school-age stutterers: A parent-child fluency group approach. *Seminars in Speech and Language, 12,* 309–322.

Kelly, E. M., & Conture, E. G. (1992). Speaking rates, response time latencies, and interrupting behaviors of young stutterers, nonstutterers, and their mothers. *Journal of Speech and Hearing Research, 35,* 1256–1267.

LaSalle, L., & Conture, E. (1995). Disfluency clusters of children who stutter: Relation of stuttering to self-repairs. *Journal of Speech, Language, and Hearing Research, 38,* 965–977.

Lincoln, M., & Onslow, M. (1997). Long-term outcome of early intervention for stuttering. *American Journal of Speech-Language Pathology, 6,* 51–58.

Manning, W. (1996). *Clinical decision making in the diagnosis and treatment of fluency disorders.* Albany, NY: Delmar Publishing.

Martin, R., Haroldson, S., & Triden, K. (1984). Stuttering and speech naturalness. *Journal of Speech and Hearing Disorders, 49,* 53–58.

Onslow, M., Andrews, C., & Lincoln, M. (1994). A control/experimental trial of an operant treatment for early stuttering. *Journal of Speech and Hearing Research, 37,* 1244–1259.

Oyler, M. E. (1996). *Vulnerability in stuttering children* (No. 9602431). Ann Arbor, MI: UMI Dissertation Services.

Oyler, M. E., & Ramig, P. R. (1995, December). *Vulnerability in stuttering children.* Seminar presented at the American Speech-Language-Hearing Association Annual Convention, Orlando, FL.

Peters, T. J., & Guitar, B. G. (1991). *Stuttering: An integrated approach to its nature and treatment.* Baltimore, MD: Williams & Wilkins.

Pindzola, R. H. (1986). A description of some selected stuttering instruments. *Journal of Childhood Communication Disorders, 9,* 183–200.

Pindzola, R. (1987). *Stuttering intervention program.* Austin, TX: Pro-Ed.

Pindzola, R. H., & White, D. (1986). A protocol for differentiating the incipient stutterer. *Language, Speech, and Hearing Services in the Schools, 17,* 2–15.

Ramig, P. R. (1993). Parent-clinician-child partnership in the therapeutic process of the preschool- and elementary-aged child who stutters. *Seminars in Speech and Language, 14,* 226–237.

Ramig, P. R., & Bennett, E. M. (1997). Clinical management of children: Direct management strategies. In R. F. Curlee & G. M. Siegel (Eds.), *Nature and treatment of stuttering* (2nd ed., pp. 292–312). Needham Heights, MA: Allyn & Bacon.

Riley, G. (1981). *Stuttering Prediction Instrument for Young Children.* Austin, TX: Pro-Ed.

Riley, G. D. (1994). *Stuttering Severity Instrument for Children and Adults* (3rd ed.). Austin, TX: Pro-Ed.

Riley, G., & Riley, J. (1982). Evaluating stuttering problems in children. *Journal of Childhood Communication Disorders, 6,* 15–25.

Rustin, L. (1987). The treatment of childhood dysfluency through active parental involvement. In L. Rustin, H. Purser, & H. Rowley (Eds.), *Progress in the treatment of fluency disorders* (pp. 168–180). London: Taylor and Francis.

Rustin, L., Botterill, W., & Kelman, E. (1996). *Assessment and therapy for young dysfluent children: Family interaction.* San Diego, CA: Singular Publishing Group.

Schulze, H., & Johannsen, H. (1991). Importance of parent-child interaction in the genesis of stuttering. *Folia Phoniatrica, 43,* 133–143.

Schwartz, H., & Conture, E. (1988). Subgrouping young stutterers: A behavioral perspective. *Journal of Speech and Hearing Research, 31,* 62–71.

Shine, R. (1980). *Systematic fluency training for young children.* Tigard, OR: C.C. Publications.

Smith, A., & Kelly, A. (1997). Stuttering: A dynamic, multifactorial model. In R. F. Curlee & G. M. Siegel (Eds.), *Nature and treatment of stuttering* (2nd ed., pp. 204–217). Needham Heights, MA: Allyn & Bacon.

Van Riper, C. (1973). *The treatment of stuttering.* Englewood Cliffs, NJ: Prentice-Hall.

Wall, M., & Myers, F. (1995). *Clinical management of childhood stuttering* (2nd ed.). Baltimore, MD: University Park Press.

Williams, D. (1971). Stuttering therapy for children. In L. Travis (Ed.), *Handbook of speech pathology* (pp. 1073–1093). New York. Appleton-Century-Crofts.

Williams, D. E. (1974). Evaluation. In C. W. Starkweather (Ed.), *Therapy for stutterers* (pp. 9–19). Memphis, TN: Speech Foundation of America.

Wingate, M. (1962). Evaluation of stuttering: II. Environmental stress and critical appraisal of speech. *Journal of Speech and Hearing Disorders, 27,* 244–257.

Yairi, E. (1997). Disfluency characteristics of childhood stuttering. In R. F. Curlee & G. M. Siegel (Eds.), *Nature and treatment of stuttering* (2nd ed., pp. 49–78). Needham Heights, MA: Allyn & Bacon.

Yairi, E., & Ambrose, N. (1992). A longitudinal study of stuttering in children: A preliminary report. *Journal of Speech and Hearing Research, 35,* 755–760.

Yairi, E., Ambrose, N., & Niermann, R. (1993). The early months of stuttering. A developmental study. *Journal of Speech and Hearing Research, 36,* 521–528.

Yaruss, S. (1997a). Clinical measurement of stuttering behaviors. *Contemporary Issues in Communication Science and Disorders, 24,* 33–44.

Yaruss, J. S. (1997b). Clinical implications of situational variability in preschool children who stutter. *Journal of Fluency Disorders, 22,* 187–203.

Yaruss, J. S., LaSalle, L. R., & Conture, E. G. (1998). Evaluating stuttering in young children: Diagnostic data. *American Journal of Speech-Language Pathology, 7,* 62–76.

Yaruss, J. S., Max, M. S., Newman, R., & Campbell, J. H. (1998). Comparing real-time and transcript-based techniques for measuring stuttering. *Journal of Fluency Disorders, 23,* 137–152.

Zebrowski, P. M. (1994). Stuttering. In J. Tomblin, H. Morris, & D. Spriestersbach (Eds.), *Diagnosis in speech-language pathology* (pp. 215–245). San Diego, CA: Singular Publishing Group.

Zebrowski, P. M., & Schum, R. (1993). Counseling parents of children who stutter. *American Journal of Speech-Language Pathology, 2,* 65–73.

3

Stuttering Prevention and Early Intervention: A Multiprocess Approach

SHERYL RIDENER GOTTWALD
C. WOODRUFF STARKWEATHER

INTRODUCTION

Although research indicates that many young children will recover from stuttering without help (e.g., Ryan, 1990; Yairi & Ambrose, 1992; Yairi, Ambrose, Paden, & Throneburg, 1996), some preschoolers will develop a confirmed and persistent stuttering problem. Early intervention for stuttering, typically provided during the child's preschool or early school-age years, has a history of success, as reported in the literature since the mid-1980s (e.g., Adams, 1992; Culp, 1984; Gregory & Hill, 1980; Lincoln, Onslow, & Reed, 1997; Shine, 1984; Starkweather, Gottwald, & Halfond, 1990). Several of these studies claim that close to 100% of the children who received treatment maintained normal fluency up to 1 year postdischarge (Culp, 1984; Meyers, 1991; Shine, 1984; Starkweather et al., 1990). An early intervention program can help youngsters avoid the lifelong stressors often associated with stuttering.

Rationale for Early Stuttering Intervention

There is widespread agreement that early intervention for young children who stutter is beneficial (Curlee & Yairi, 1997). For example, Culp (1984) described the outcomes for seven children who participated in her Preschool Fluency Development Program. Six of these children reportedly continued to maintain normal fluency 2 years post-treatment. Results reported by Starkweather et al. (1990) indicated that the 29 children who completed their early intervention program maintained normal fluency up to 2 years after discharge from treatment. Shine (1984) reported that 13 of the 14 preschoolers who participated in his Fluency Training Program maintained fluency during follow-up visits scheduled between 1 to 5 years post-treatment. Lincoln and Onslow (1997) reported results of a long-term outcome study. Preschool children and their families participated in The Lidcombe Program, a parent-administered early intervention program for stuttering. The near-zero levels of stuttering that were reported when the children were discharged from treatment were maintained up to 7 years post-treatment.

Research in stuttering onset and development is identifying factors which place a young child at greater risk for continuing to stutter (Yairi et al., 1996). Some of those risk factors involve variables such as a family history of stuttering and the child's gender, with males being four to five times more likely to continue to stutter than females. Other variables are related to the child's growth and development; children who continue to stutter are more likely also to have other developmental problems such as speech and language difficulties (Guitar, 1998). Variables relating directly to the child's stuttering may also be predictive of stuttering persistence. The longer the child stutters and the more severe the stuttering, the more likely it is that the child will continue to stutter without intervention (Starkweather & Gottwald, 1993).

Determining the number of risk factors present is the first step in identifying children whose stuttering is unlikely to remit spontaneously. However, it is still difficult to predict with any certainty which children will recover spontaneously and which will not. If a child continues to stutter because interventions have not been initiated early enough, the outcome may be the development of a speech disorder with the potential to hurt the child throughout his or her life. Since early intervention for stuttering is effective and usually conducted over a relatively short period, and since involvement in therapy will not harm a child or family (Starkweather, 1997), we feel that the decision to treat any preschooler who is stuttering is strongly supported.

There is a range of options available for intervening with the young child who stutters. These treatment choices may include involvement in a comprehensive and intensive treatment program, participation in a series of parent counseling sessions, telephone counseling plus educational readings, and child participation in a fluency enhancement group. Applying a risk-benefit analysis when making decisions about intervention, as recommended by Bernstein Ratner (1997), allows the clinician to weigh the likelihood that the child will recover spontaneously against the limitations that involvement in a treatment program might impose.

The Multiprocess Stuttering Prevention and Early Intervention Program

In the intervention program described here, the child's speech patterns and communicative environment are modified simultaneously to produce rapid and long-lasting changes in the child's fluency. Improvement in speech fluency for young children who stutter has been repeatedly described in the literature when environmental modifications have been implemented (e.g., Langlois & Long, 1988; Manning, 1996; Rustin, 1987; Wall & Myers, 1995), when the child's speech patterns are directly modified (e.g., Ingham, 1993; Onslow, Andrews, & Lincoln, 1994; Shine, 1984), and when both variables are addressed concurrently (e.g., Gottwald & Starkweather, 1995; Gregory & Hill, 1980; Zebrowski, 1997).

This "multiprocess" method is based on the premise that stuttering develops when the child lacks the capacity to speak as fluently as the environment demands. This Demands and Capacities model has been described in detail elsewhere (Adams, 1990; Starkweather & Givens-Ackerman, 1997; Starkweather & Gottwald, 1990). The child's developing fluency skill results from the meshing of the child's growing capacities with environmental events that challenge the use of those capacities.

Capacities for Fluent Speech Production

Starkweather (1987) has suggested that fluent speech is produced continuously, at a rapid rate, and with minimal effort. To demonstrate this skill, young children develop competencies in several areas. They need adequate speech motor control to coarticulate smoothly, rapidly, and with minimal effort. They need mastery of language formulation and production skills. They need to be able to express syntactically complex and lengthy sentences, retrieve from an ever-increasing vocabulary store, and use language to accomplish a variety of tasks, including asserting and questioning. They need to learn to function independently, tolerate stress, and function within the behavioral guidelines established for them. From a cognitive perspective, fluency will be supported when children are able to solve problems, plan, and remember consequences. These capacities for fluency typically mature during the child's preschool and early school years.

Demands on Fluency

As a child's capacities for fluency are growing, so too are the demands for fluency, conditions imposed by the listener or by the child that may stress developing fluency skills. The speech behaviors of significant people in the child's life may be one of those demanding variables. For example, research has demonstrated that children with more advanced stuttering had parents who talked much more quickly than their children (Kelly, 1994; Yaruss & Conture, 1995). If the child who is at risk for stuttering attempts to imitate that faster parental rate but does not have the motoric ability to do so, fluency may be compromised. Likewise, other studies have indicated that mothers of children who stuttered spoke faster than mothers of children who did not stutter (Meyers & Freeman, 1985a; Yaruss & Conture, 1995) and asked more questions than mothers of nonstuttering children (Meyers, 1990). Kloth, Janssen, Kraaimaat, and Brutten (1995), in a longitudinal study of children genetically at risk for developing stuttering, found that the children who did not develop confirmed stuttering spoke more slowly than those who did eventually stutter. Other speech behaviors that clinicians may find useful to examine include the kind and number of questions parents ask and the amount of time parents spend in conversations with their children.

Demands may also be identified in family interaction patterns. Meyers and Freeman (1985b) presented data that indicated that mothers interrupted children more when the children stuttered. Likewise, the children in that study were more disfluent when interrupting other speakers and when being interrupted. Kelly and Conture (1992) demonstrated that stuttering was more likely to occur with "simultalk," that is, when both the child and parent spoke at the same time. When Winslow and Guitar (1994) encouraged a family to apply clear turn-taking rules, the child demonstrated decreased stuttering. If a child plays a more assertive role in interaction with the parents, fluency may also be compromised (Weiss & Zebrowski, 1992). Topic initiation, too, has been correlated with disfluency (Bell, 1986). Other interaction variables that might impact a child's fluency levels include parental requests for verbal performance and the pace of conversational interchanges with the child.

Family reactions to stuttering may be demanding of fluency. Negative comments, such as "stop stuttering," or instructions to speak otherwise (e.g., "slow down"; "take a deep breath") tell children convincingly that the way they are currently talking is not acceptable. In an effort to compensate for the time stuttering occupies, children are likely to struggle and force their way through a stuttering episode, further complicating the speech problem. Some families express feelings of fear and frustration regarding the child's stuttering nonverbally. They may freeze their body position at the moment of stuttering, turn away from the child, or look worriedly at the child who is stuttering. In addition to conveying to children that their speech is undesirable, these nonverbal reactions may also convey pain and discomfort. While struggling to avoid stuttering, children may also be grappling with guilt resulting from feeling that they have caused their parents discomfort. Families that engage in "the conspiracy of silence"—pretending, when their child stutters, that nothing is happening—may send the child a message that stuttering is profoundly shameful.

Family lifestyle characteristics may be demanding developing fluency skill, especially when those characteristics affect the rate at which activities are completed or the tension levels involved in completion of these activities. Children whose lives are filled with things to do, and whose families are continuously rushing from one activity to the next, may communicate in a similar fashion. To fit in talking, their rate of speech may be rapid and the time between turns minimal. If expectations for performance are high, anxiety may be heightened and tension levels overall may be raised, making it more difficult for children to manage their speech mechanism.

A final area of demand for fluency that is noteworthy here is uneven development of the skills (language, speech, motor, cognition) that contribute to fluent speech. For example, if preschoolers demonstrate precocious language skills, they may attempt to produce long, complex, assertive language ideas at a young age. If their speech motor skills are not as advanced as their language skills, those speech motor skills may not be able to support their language skills. It is possible that this mismatch between developmental levels may of itself be demanding of developing fluency.

As explained earlier, we believe that some form of intervention should be initiated when demands outweigh capacities and fluency breaks down. As suggested by Zebrowski (1997) and others (e.g., Bernstein-Ratner, 1997), we concur that the nature and intensiveness of the treatment program will vary depending on individual needs. The program described here is a multiprocess one, involving direct therapy components for children and their families as well as small group opportunities for both parents and children. Families may participate in one or more of these components based on the number of risk factors present as well as on the family's feelings about the child's speech. The goal of intervention is to prevent the development and habituation of more advanced stuttering behaviors by intervening as soon as possible after stuttering onset.

THE PROGRAM

Assessment

The purpose of assessment is to evaluate the child's capacities for fluency and to identify demands that might be stressing those capacities. The clinician collects this information in a variety of ways, including examining typical interactions of the child with family, teachers, and peers; interviewing significant people in the child's life; and working directly with the child to manipulate fluency levels. In all of these diagnostic contexts, the clinician collects information about the presence of risk factors that increase the likelihood that the child will continue to stutter.

Collecting Information Prior to the Evaluation

The initial telephone contact is an opportune time for the clinician to learn about the child's and family's speech patterns and to begin providing suggestions for intervention. Since stuttering may develop rapidly, the opportunity to intervene early may reverse or at least slow the development of struggled speech. Further, parents are often quite distraught when they make their first contact with a speech-language pathologist. When they have an opportunity to express their worries during that first telephone contact and when a professional provides some concrete suggestions for remediation, those feelings of concern are somewhat mitigated. We have found that, when telephone counseling is effective, later therapy time is reduced.

Following the initial telephone contact, the clinician sends case history and observation forms to the child's family. Parents send back written permission for the clinician to contact other important people in the child's life, including teachers and day-care staff. The contributions of these people to the diagnostic process are invaluable as they provide information about the child's speech outside the home setting.

Interviewing the Family and Preschool Staff

During the parent interview, the clinician collects information that will help identify the presence or absence of risk factors for stuttering persistence. The acquisition of a basic case history provides information about the occurrence of stuttering in the child's family and the child's speech, language, motor, and cognitive development. A history of the child's stuttering problem identifies factors such as duration of stuttering, the development of secondary behaviors, and changes in the child's reactivity.

During the interview the clinician also seeks to identify potential demands as well as the family's need for information and support. When parents feel guilty, they will find it more difficult to address the child's problem. The interview provides an opportunity to explore reactions of family members and others to the child's stuttering. In this way, the clinician identifies who might benefit from higher levels of emotional support and who might be more actively involved in the intervention process from the outset of the intervention.

Information about the child's typical daily and weekly routines may pinpoint areas of demand for fluency. In an attempt to provide the most that they can for their children, parents sometimes schedule numerous activities throughout the week. The family then spends much time rushing from one thing to the next, leaving minimal time for quality interaction. It is easy to see how fluency can be compromised with this kind of lifestyle.

During the interview parents are asked to talk about any stressful or exciting life events that may have occurred at the onset of the stuttering or at any point in which they noticed changes in the child's speech patterns. Although we cannot say for certain that a direct relationship existed between the child's stuttering and the event, we may begin to extract meaningful similarities. For example, if the parents reported increased stuttering in September when the child began preschool, in December when the child began a holiday vacation, and in June when the child began summer vacation, it might be hypothesized that times of transition disrupt this child's fluency.

Discipline is often an area of concern for parents whose children stutter. Sometimes parents report that stuttering increases when the child is disciplined, and parents may then avoid disciplining the child to eliminate the risk of more stuttering. Without consistent management, the child's behavior may become more problematic and the stuttering may be indirectly reinforced.

It is also important to ask families about the child's strengths. When the family is upset about the child's speech problem, the focus is on the stuttering rather than on the child as a person with a variety of skills. Talking about the child's interests and things the child excels in will help put the speech problem in perspective.

Teacher and day-care staff interviews provide additional information about environmental characteristics that have an impact on the child's stuttering. Preschool teachers may be able to identify specific activities that are associated with increases or decreases in stuttering. If a child is more fluent during structured activities in which responses are more predictable and routine (weather, calendar) but has more difficulty during free choice activities, conversation structure may prove to be an important variable. Teachers and day-care staff may also provide information about the child's peer interactions and the reactions of peers to the child's speech.

Collecting Speech Samples for Analysis

To conduct direct assessments of the speech, language, and communication behaviors of the child and the significant people in the child's life, videotaped samples of interactions in at least two but preferably three different contexts should be collected. When possible, transcribed samples from videotapes of the child playing at home with family members and interacting at school or day-care with staff and peers should be used as the basis for formal analysis. When planning for these videotape sessions, we encourage families and teachers to make the interaction as natural as possible, since that provides the most realistic picture of the child's fluency skills.

Utterances that are largely intelligible and consecutive are utilized for fluency measurement. We recommend transcribing at least 25 utterances produced by each significant person in the child's life. We also transcribe at least 25 utterances produced by the child in at least two but preferably three different interaction situations, providing 300–500 syllables per interaction.

Measuring Speech and Interactions of Significant Others

The clinician may choose to evaluate the speech characteristics of both parents in a two-parent family or only of the parent who is the primary caregiver. If the child attends preschool or daycare, or has a live-in nanny, the clinician may wish to assess the speech of the person who spends the most time with the child.

After the sample is transcribed, the clinician assesses the continuity of the adult's speech by highlighting and counting the presence of discontinuities. Rate of fluent speech is measured in 10 consecutive utterances that are of relatively equal length. The rate measures are then compared to normative speech rate measures reported elsewhere in the literature (e.g., Amster, 1984; Kowal, O'Connell, & Sabin, 1975).

In addition to these measures, the clinician examines the number of questions the adult asks and the nature of those questions. If the child is asked to answer many questions that require extensive language formulation and expression, fluency may be compromised. Similarly, if the adult makes frequent requests of the child to perform verbally, such as, "Tell me what your teacher said about the field trip," the stress of having to remember facts, organize ideas, choose appropriate language, and perform for an adult may precipitate fluency breakdown.

Since research has shown a relationship between children's stuttering and interruptions (e.g., Kelly & Conture, 1992; Meyers & Freeman, 1985b; Winslow & Guitar, 1994), we measure the amount of time the adult spoke at the same time as the child. This talking overlap time is measured in seconds with a stop watch. In addition, we measure overall talking time for the adult and then compare that with the percentage of time that the child talked in the interaction. If the adult monopolizes the conversation, pressure to communicate may be increased as the child attempts to interject his or her own ideas. On the other hand, if the parent rarely contributes to the interaction, the responsibility for shaping the conversation rests with the child, which may also prove demanding of fluency.

The clinician examines the reactions of others to the child's speech and stuttering. Verbal comments directly related to stuttering are recorded, and nonverbal responses, such as facial expressions or body movements, are identified. Likewise, it is often useful to count the frequency with which accepting and nonaccepting comments occur in the adult's speech sample. Shames and Florence (1980) described a method that readers may find useful for coding positive and negative statements made by parents.

Observing the way in which parents and teachers structure and participate in the child's play will provide information about how much responsibility the child assumes in these interactions. Adults who are able to help the child identify a play theme and who facilitate the child's exploration of that theme will foster a more relaxed and organized experience, which in the end will minimize tension and anxiety. If, on the other hand, adults introduce numerous play topics and move quickly from one idea to the next without clarifying the child's role in that play, anxiety levels may quickly rise. That anxiety may be translated into increased muscle tension, which may then be expressed as stuttering.

Parents and teachers frequently report that when children are being reprimanded, periods of stuttering increase in both frequency and severity. So it is useful to ask adults to talk about the behavior management methods they prefer, how successful they feel those methods have been, and the impact, if any, of their behavior management strategies on the child's fluency.

Finally, it is helpful to examine the child's fluency levels while playing with siblings and peers. The child may feel more relaxed interacting with a younger sibling and thus fluency skills may be more resistant to breakdown. However, the competition may be increased when the child interacts with siblings or peers closer in age, and tension levels may rise as the children vie for leadership and attention. This increased tension may contribute to increases in stuttering.

Analyzing the Child's Speech, Language, and Fluency Skills

First, the fluent syllables produced by the child are counted. The clinician notes how effortful the child's fluent speech sounded and measures rate of fluent speech. The number and kind of normal disfluencies are also counted.

Next, the clinician computes the frequency and severity of the stuttering events that occurred. The types of discontinuities are noted on the transcription and the frequency of occurrence per total syllables is determined. In addition, the frequency of occurrence for each type of discontinuity is computed for total syllables stuttered. Children with higher percentages of prolongations and blocks may demonstrate increased levels of muscle tension. This may affect both their prognosis for remediation and the methods of intervention that are chosen.

We measure the duration of each of the child's stuttering episodes with a stopwatch. The total time the child spends speaking is also measured, and the percentage of disfluent speech time (PDST) is calculated. The PDST provides a measure of the proportion of speaking time that is taken up by stuttering.

The average number of iterations per stuttering event is calculated for part-word and monosyllabic word repetitions. The rate and rhythm of these repetitions are informally assessed; rapid and irregular repetitions may indicate a more advanced stuttering problem. The presence of muscle tension during stuttering further contributes to an estimate of stuttering severity. The occurrence of pitch rise, vocal tremors and quivers (disrhythmic phonation), and alterations in volume during moments of disfluency are indicative of increased tension and more advanced stuttering.

Likewise, the clinician notes the occurrence of secondary features, as they may be signs that, on some level, the child is actively trying to "escape" or "avoid" stuttering (Guitar, 1998). Some young children we have seen have pushed their hand against their cheeks in an attempt to "push out the sound." Other body movements young children have used in their attempts to struggle past a difficult word included jumping up and down, striking their jaw or head, stamping their feet, and walking around in circles. Recently the mother of a 3-year-old told the first author about how her son had discovered the use of starter words to avoid stuttering. The mother was asking her son to take his time to tell her a story and he responded with, "It's okay, Mom, if I just say, 'You know' first, then I won't have bumpy speech."

Finally, a formal stuttering measurement device such as the Stuttering Severity Instrument–3 (Riley, 1994) is administered, to compare the child's stuttering with that of a representative group of children who stutter. The Systematic Disfluency Analysis (Hill & Campbell, 1987) provides a detailed inventory of stuttering types, and the Stocker Probe Technique (Stocker, 1980) examines the effects of utterance length and complexity as well as pragmatic complexity on speech continuity.

Next, the clinician works directly with the child to assess the variability of the child's fluency with changes in the child's speaking environment. The clinician begins by providing a fluency enhancing environment during play with the child. Some components of a fluency enhancing model (FEM) (Starkweather et al., 1990) are:

- Slow-normal rate of speech
- Short, simple sentences
- Numerous pauses and silences
- Reduced demands for nonspontaneous speech
- Slow and relaxed conversation pace
- Use of disfluencies that are normal for child's age
- Elimination of questions requiring long, complex answers.

The characteristics of this FEM will vary from child to child, depending on the perceived demands noted in the child's family and school interactions. For example, if it was noted that the parent or teacher spoke rapidly but that the child's speech was noticeably slower, so one characteristic of the fluency enhancing model would be use of a slower rate of speech by the clinician.

It is helpful to assess the child's awareness of and reaction to stuttering and to speaking in general. Very young children experiencing stuttering may already have some strong negative feelings about talking. Following periods of stuttering, children have said "I can't talk" or "I can't say my words," expressing frustration and anxiety. Other preschoolers have said that they "hate talking" and "will never learn to talk good"; these are expressions of feelings of anger and hopelessness that we tend to associate more with people who have stuttered over a long term and not with preschoolers.

The clinician might begin the process of assessing the child's awareness of and feelings about the stuttering by pseudo-stuttering in the course of conversation with the child. If there is no reaction to the clinician's stuttering, the clinician might pseudo-stutter again and comment nonchalantly about it ("Sometimes I have bumpy speech"). Often if children are aware of having speech difficulty, they will tell the clinician that they have bumpy speech, too. This provides the clinician with an opportunity to begin talking about stuttering with the child in a reassuring and supportive way, using words that the child will understand. For the child, this speech difficulty will no longer be something so horrible that no one can talk about it.

The evaluation includes assessment of phonology, language, motor, cognitive, and social-emotional development. An inventory of the child's articulation skills at the word and connected speech levels provides information about speech sounds the child has not yet mastered and about the child's coarticulation abilities.

Language measures are utilized to assess the semantic and syntactic complexity of the child's sample. Research has demonstrated that stuttering is associated with language complexity (Watkins & Yairi, 1997). Type-token ratios provide a rough estimate of semantic complexity, and the clinician also observes the child's word-finding skills. Mean length of utterance is calculated and the frequency of utterances containing embedded or conjoined elements noted. The child's pragmatic skills are also analyzed. Topic initiations and assertive statements are counted, as those two pragmatic functions have been found to be related to the occurrence of stuttering.

The clinician observes and informally assesses development in other areas that may be associated with fluency skill. The speed and agility with which children move their bodies in space provides some information about gross motor development. Finger manipulation for tasks such as zippering, coloring, or building with blocks provides information about fine motor skills. Likewise, an oral-peripheral examination including testing of diadochokinesis assesses oral and speech motor skill. The child's play level, ability to attend to a play theme, and ability to solve problems gives the diagnostic team information about cognitive development. Social-emotional development is informally assessed by observing such things as the child's interaction and negotiation skills, level of independence, and ability to tolerate frustration.

Once the adult and child samples have been analyzed separately, they are compared to evaluate the degree to which the adult models match the child's capacity levels. The larger the discrepancy between adult and child performance levels, the greater the demand on the child's fluency skills. Although we do not have normative data, we calculate relative measures which indicate the degree of difference between the child and the adult on identified variables. Large discrepancies provide "red flags" for the clinician to consider the probability that a particular variable may be fluency demanding.

When we provide feedback about the assessment process to the child's family, we begin by describing the child's fluency, speech, and language capacities. We then talk about specific environmental factors that we feel are supporting fluency and would benefit from continuation. Likewise, we discuss environmental factors that if altered for a period of time may enhance fluency. Families and teachers are repeatedly told that the interaction patterns they use now are not wrong or inferior, but really quite normal. We tell families that the alterations we ask them to make will not need to be permanent ones; once the child's fluency levels have increased, and capacities and demands are no longer discrepant, families and teachers can once again move back to more familiar and typical interactions. We encourage families and teachers to ask questions at this point in the evaluation process. We are careful not to provide too much information in this first session, as that can be overwhelming. Originally we found ourselves saying the same things to parents session after session. It soon became apparent that this occurred because we sometimes provided information before parents were ready to process it.

Families and teachers are provided with one or two techniques that they might try at home or in school to decrease the effects of suspected demands. For example, adults may be asked to pause for 2 seconds before responding to the child's requests. This will slow the pace of the conversation if time pressure is a suspected demand.

Intervention

This multiprocess intervention program is designed to (a) reduce demands on the child's current level of fluency, which may stem from the environment or from the child, and (b) enhance the child's capacities for producing fluent speech.

Our treatment plans are individualized and evolve as the child and his or her environment changes. Although the family constellation usually provides the focus for intervention, the child's interactions with preschool or day-care staff and with peers must be considered an integral part of the therapy plan. The significant adults, including parents and teachers, participate in counseling sessions where they learn to identify and modify potential fluency stressors. The children work individually with the clinician to modify speech behaviors through the use of imagery, modeling, and reinforcement. As the child's fluency skills are strengthened, interactions with peers both in and outside the clinic are scheduled to facilitate transfer and maintenance of fluency skills.

If an intensive intervention program is initiated, sessions are scheduled on a weekly basis. The child participates in an hour of individual therapy at least once a week, while the child's family also meets with the clinician for a 60-minute session on a weekly basis. If the child attends a preschool or day-care program, additional intervention sessions may be scheduled in that environment to work directly with the child and to educate the child's caregivers. As the child's stuttering decreases, small group intervention sessions may replace individual treatment, and sessions are gradually scheduled on a less frequent basis.

Intervening With the Child's Family, Preschool, and Neighborhood

It is important to keep in mind that a child grows and develops in the context of a family system. The behaviors of one member of the family directly affect the responses of the other members. This family system interacts with other systems, including the neighborhood and the child's preschool. These systems have been functioning in a largely successful way long before the family sought help. If we try to change the system without active involvement of all of its members, we most likely will fail. That is why each family's intervention plan is individualized and the members of all of the systems of which the child is a member are integrally involved in developing the plan. They are the experts when it comes to understanding how their systems work. If we choose not to utilize that knowledge, it is likely that the system will not change and the child's fluency skills may continue to be negatively impacted.

The process we use when working with parents and teachers has multiple steps. We begin by debriefing, asking the adult to comment about anything related to the child's speech that occurred since the last session. In this way successes and problems are identified. Next, the adult and clinician choose a focus for the session. For example, if during debriefing the parents talked about the interruptions they noticed in family interactions, the clinician might ask the parents if they would like to discuss management of interruptions in the current session.

Once a target is chosen, the adult and clinician brainstorm ways to address the target. We encourage families and teachers to make a written list of the ways in which the target might be managed. Families and school staff then examine the potential strategies to choose the one best suited to them.

Once a strategy has been chosen, the adult practices using the strategy first alone with the clinician and then with the child and clinician. This practice time provides parents and teachers with an opportunity to try a particular technique and receive immediate feedback. When both the parent or teacher and the clinician feel satisfied with the newly learned technique, the significant adults will try the technique at home or school and report about its success in future sessions.

Providing Accurate Information.   When asked to listen to their own speech, many adults are surprised to discover that normally fluent speech contains disfluencies that speakers use to gain formulation time. It is beneficial to identify and provide examples of normal disfluencies, such as relaxed whole word and phrase repetitions, filled and unfilled pauses, and sentence revisions.

In addition, parents learn about symptoms that may indicate that the stuttering problem is developing in severity. If they know that prolongations with pitch rise indicate increased tension and struggle, they can initiate modifications that may reduce the demands supporting this reaction. Also, when the child is in the maintenance phase of therapy, knowledge about signs of risk will help parents know when more active intervention might be beneficial.

Parents and teachers may need information about factors that maintain stuttering in some children. We stress that not all of these factors are important for each family. However, with this information, parents and teachers are better observers outside the clinic setting. Other components of this educational phase of therapy include describing the treatment components of the multiprocess program, defining relapse, and developing methods for managing regression if it occurs.

Learning New Ways to Talk. If parents or teachers speak with a rate of speech that is much faster than the child's rate, the child may try to match that rate to maintain the pace of the conversation that the adult has set up. Attempting to speak more quickly than the motor speech system can manage may precipitate fluency breakdown.

Parents and teachers can learn to use a slower rate of speech, closer to the rate used by their children. When adults pause more often, use shorter sentences, and move more slowly as they talk, speech rate generally decreases. Adults might listen to an audiotape of their child's speech to perceive how slowly the child is actually talking.

Along with reducing their rates of speech, parents and teachers might also slow down the pace of the conversation. In a typical conversation, speakers allow no more than 1 second to elapse before someone else begins talking. We have found that, if parents allow more time between conversational turns, the pressure to communicate and the tension associated with that pressure are reduced. We recommend that parents and teachers use the "2-second pause." That is, they pause for approximately 2 seconds before answering or responding to the child's utterances. This slows the pace of conversation considerably, eliminates interruptions by the adult, and tells the child that there is ample time to formulate and express ideas.

Verbal performance on demand is often a difficult task for children who stutter. We recommend that parents and teachers modify their expectations for language use by children who are showing signs of stuttering. One strategy adults might implement in this regard involves substituting comments for questions. Parents are often surprised to see how easy it is to get children to talk about experiences by parent modeling and self-talk rather than through questioning. Because the message the child shares is spontaneous, the time pressure to communicate is reduced and the message is more likely to be produced with normal fluency. If questions are asked, it is recommended that parents used closed-ended requests requiring the child to produce a simple answer in response.

Language demands may also be expressed in the sheer amount of talking that occurs in a home or school setting. If interaction is valued and occurs frequently, the child may attempt to talk as often as the other speakers. However, it may take more time and effort for the child to formulate and express language ideas; the child may feel pressured to keep talking but not be able to keep up. In our experience, this occurs in homes where parents are teachers or speech-language pathologists! These families appeared to spend more time talking, and the level of language is often advanced. We recommend that overall talking time be reduced. We assure parents that children will not suffer any adverse effects if the amount of talking in a family decreases.

There are several language-based demands that we have found to be pertinent for some children. When some children communicate a message, their anxiety increases until the recipient of the message confirms that they have understood the child's intent. Often, these children will repeat their message more insistently until the listener responds in some way. Usually the repetitions contain disfluencies as the child's anxiety and tension increase. We encourage parents and teachers to let children know that they have been heard, even when a direct response may not be required.

To introduce a new idea, a child has to develop and formulate the idea, retrieve appropriate vocabulary and grammar, and plan and execute the speech act. In addition to the cognitive, semantic, syntactic, and motor demands of such a task, children must also manage the associated pragmatic demands. They must be skilled at getting and keeping the listener's attention, meeting the language needs of the listener, and knowing how to repair the conversation should breakdown occur. The anxiety that such added pressure may stimulate may be expressed in increased muscle tension and stuttering. If, however, the parent scaffolds the conversation, providing structure for the interchange, responsibility for the success of the interchange is at least shared, if not assumed entirely by the adult. Tension that might result from uncertainty about the successful transmission of a message is thus reduced and the child is more likely to speak with ease.

If interruptions occur in an interaction, the pace of the conversation is increased. The child may feel pressured to communicate the message quickly before someone else takes over. Reducing this time pressure may enhance the child's ability to speak fluently. When a family establishes clear turn-taking rules, children know that they will have a turn to talk and that they will not have to compete to get that turn. Tension levels are thus reduced and fluent speech production is enhanced.

Some families have resorted to using objects, such as passing the salt shaker around at the dinner table, to indicate who holds the conversation floor at any particular time. Some families have set up quiet times during more stressful talking periods. If children stutter more as they compete for their parents' attention while preparing a meal or getting ready for an outing, that is probably not an ideal interaction time. Parents may identify these more stressful periods as "quiet times" where talking is kept to a minimum. Children can be directed to noninteractive activities such as watching a favorite video, playing a computer game, reading, or coloring.

Families can identify special interaction times where the parent and child who stutters spend some uninterrupted play time together. Parents are advised to set aside a 15- to 30-minute play period with the child each day, where interruptions are minimized and the parent can focus on setting up a more ideal communication environment. Children seem to look forward to this relaxed interaction and the individual attention they receive from the parent. Parents feel more justified in eliminating talking at stressful times when they know they have this special interaction period scheduled at another time in the day.

Modifying the General Communicative Environment.   Some families have found it helpful to schedule ample time for each daily activity. When children are rushing from one activity to the next, time pressure is increased and fluency may be sacrificed. If the pace of activity is reduced, tension is also lessened and the accomplishment of any motor task, including speaking, is made easier. In an attempt to adjust the daily schedule, several parents decided to get up 30 minutes earlier each morning, to allow more time to prepare for the day. Other families reduced the number of the children's activities so that they could move at a more leisurely pace.

When children encounter surprises or unexpected events, excitement and associated increases in overall body tension result. This tension, even when positive, may be transferred directly to the child's speech muscles and then precipitate fluency breakdown. When parents and teachers schedule a predictable daily routine, the child knows what to expect, and anxiety that may result from the unknown is reduced. Likewise, adequate preparation for changes in that routine is also recommended. Using weekly calendars, talking about changes several days in advance, and involving the child in planning for changes will reduce the uncertainty that sometimes accompanies the unfamiliar.

Discipline can sometimes precipitate increases in stuttering. Some families allow their children to explain why they engaged in the misdeed or ask their children to tell why they are being punished. Both approaches require extensive formulation (the children must figure out a way to convince the adult that they really haven't misbehaved!) at a time when tension levels are significantly increased. It is easy to see why stuttering might result. We recommend that parents set up discipline methods that do not require input from the child. Instead, the adult tells the child in simple terms what the misdeed was and what the punishment will be. The child is not allowed to talk during this period or to discuss the incident when the punishment is concluded.

When a child stutters, the speech problem often becomes the focus of attention. The child experiences failure when talking, and adult discussion about the child revolves around how much stuttering there was on any particular day. It is helpful, though, to keep the child's speech difficulties in some perspective. There are most likely many other things the child excels in, and providing opportunities for the child to engage in those areas of strength would be helpful. For example, one family realized how much their child enjoyed swimming. They enrolled him in a team at the local YMCA, and he became the star swimmer for the team. This accomplishment, rather than the child's speech problem, is now the topic of discussion at family gatherings. In our view, a person's level of confidence has a direct effect on general motor control and coordination. For some children, improving self-confidence can play a large role in supporting normal fluency.

Engaging the child in manageable speech tasks is beneficial. If the child is having a particularly disfluent day, asking for an account of the day at preschool is probably too demanding a task. The parent could ask yes/no or single-word response questions instead. Children are thus able to share information in a way that supports rather than stresses current fluency levels.

Exploring Feelings and Modifying Reactions to Stuttering.   Stuttering, like any difficulty a child experiences, precipitates feelings even in the youngest of children. We have worked with 2½ year old youngsters who stamped their feet, cried and gave up trying to talk when experiencing fluency breakdown. Other preschoolers have said that they could "never talk right," that the words "just get stuck," and that "there is a monster in my throat." Feelings of anger, fear, and unworthiness may impede the child's ability to learn to use normal fluency. Furthermore, if those feelings are not acknowledged, the child may assume that the feelings and the behaviors that precipitated them are undesirable or bad. With attempts to mask the feelings or avoid the stuttering, tension levels are increased, which then increases the likelihood of stuttering.

Parents and teachers are encouraged to talk openly about the child's speech problem in words the child can understand. When the child stamps his foot in anger at not being able to produce a word, the adult might say, "That was a tough word for you. Sometimes when I have trouble talking, it makes me mad, too." The adult might then reassure the child, reflecting that we all have trouble sometimes. The adult should also let the child know that, regardless of speech difficulty, the adult always enjoys talking with and listening to the child.

Many parents have told us that they tried to ignore the child's stuttering prior to seeking help. They hoped that, by not calling attention to the child's speech, the problem would disappear. Unfortunately, some children learn instead that stuttering is too shameful to mention. Others may come to believe that their stuttering is not fully audible to others. It is beneficial to encourage parents to explore their worries in an open and accepting environment. Parents may be initially embarrassed when they realize how much they dislike listening to their child's stuttering or how upset they are to have to deal with this problem. Once these feelings and attitudes have been validated, anxiety is usually reduced.

An example may be illustrative here. After talking for several weeks about her child's stuttering, one mother realized how difficult it was for her even to say the word "stuttering." As we explored those feelings further, the mother discovered how appalled she was every time she heard her child stutter. We agreed that it was difficult to listen to a child who was struggling to talk.

As the mother's anxiety about her feelings dissipated, we were then able to help her evaluate how her feelings might be expressed when she interacted with the child. During videotape analysis, this mother learned that she often turned away, interrupted, or changed the subject when her child stuttered, behaviors indicative of the mother's need to avoid stuttering. We desensitized the mother to the child's stuttering by listening to and evaluating the child's stuttering together on videotape. The mother was then able to systematically replace some of her negative reactions with behaviors more supportive of fluency growth for her child. She learned to remain facing the child, to wait patiently until the child completed the message, to use the 2-second pause before responding to the child, and to wait for topic closure before introducing a new idea, regardless of the child's fluency levels.

Intervening With the Child in the Clinic

Working With the Child Who Is Excessively Disfluent But Shows Little Struggle. These children typically produce many whole and part-word repetitions, often with more than two iterations per disfluency episode. The repetitions are usually relaxed and rhythmic. Syllable structure is maintained and pitch levels are stable.

The first objective in working with any child who is at risk for stuttering is to set up a clinical environment that is conducive to normal fluency. The components of a fluency enhancing model (FEM) were described earlier in this chapter. Not every child will benefit from each of these suggestions. For example, some children benefit more when the clinician follows the child's conversation lead. That strategy would then be an important component of the child's FEM. However, other children become overwhelmed and more disfluent when they feel responsible for the direction of the conversation. These children are more fluent when the clinician participates in structuring the conversation by providing "scaffolds" for the child to participate more easily in the interaction. Scaffolding would then be a critical element in the child's FEM.

If the child is attempting to speak at a faster rate than feasible, the mismatch in effort and ability level may contribute to fluency breakdown. Assisting the child to use a more appropriate speech rate would then facilitate production of more continuous speech. First, the clinician will model speech produced at the target rate for the child. Pause times would be slightly exaggerated in duration. The clinician will not only model slowed speech rate, but also move more slowly overall. The pace of the session will be relaxed and sufficient time will be allowed to transition slowly from one activity to another.

The clinician may also want to describe slow speech in concrete terms. With some children we have called the slower speech "dinosaur speech" or "snail speech," matching their understanding of the concept "slow" with an image that is meaningful to them. We then move about the room like dinosaurs or snails in an exaggerated and slow-motion way. Labeling the rapid speech rate is also useful. Terms we have found to be meaningful include "rabbit speech," "jet speech," and "fire engine speech," all labels children helped us develop.

We begin by providing opportunities for the child to use the new speech rate in short, structured utterances with low propositional impact. Children use "snail speech" to label pictures attached to "fish" they have pulled out of the "lake," to describe actions on cards during a memory game, and to describe pictures in a favorite storybook. As the child becomes more skilled with rate control, the length and complexity of the utterances she produces are increased, as are the pragmatic demands. Rate control skills are transferred to more spontaneous play activities, first in a confined area such as at the table having a tea party. Once the child is successful over time at this level of play, control of space, play toys, and playmates is gradually transferred to the child.

Some children use changes in volume as a fluency strategy. The concept of an "indoor voice," as used in many preschool classrooms, is also an appropriate talking time rule at home. Children and parents can experiment with "indoor" and "outdoor" voices in the clinic and can then practice using an "indoor" voice for progressively longer periods at home.

Even some very young children in our experience have been quite disturbed by their speech difficulties. They have told us that they feel badly that they cannot talk like other people. One child said that he did not want to ever talk again. During direct therapy, we acknowledge the child's speech difficulties in words the child will understand. We tell them that at times it is hard to talk and that adults have trouble sometimes, too. We reassure them that they are learning new talking skills and that soon talking will be easier for them.

We balance discussions about speech difficulties with many opportunities for children to engage in activities they enjoy. Whenever possible, we provide children with positive feedback about their accomplishments. We also continuously remind the children how much we enjoy playing and talking with them, regardless of their fluency.

Working With Preschoolers Who Stutter and Show Signs of Struggle.   If children are having difficulty moving their speech mechanism because of stuttering, it is not surprising that they will increase muscle effort in an attempt to escape from the unpleasant feelings that stuttering precipitates. Children we have worked with have puffed air in their cheeks, squeezed their eyes shut, and protruded their tongues to produce speech. Others have tapped their leg, stamped their foot, and jumped up and down as they struggled through talking. Still others have stopped talking altogether or started to cry when their speech struggles became overwhelming.

If struggle behaviors are apparent, the first goal of therapy is to reduce the negative reactions that lead to speech struggle. Together, the child and clinician can find labels to describe the child's normally fluent and stuttered speech. Sometimes the clinician might suggest possible names based on the kind of stuttering the child has, but children often are able to label the disfluent speech. A very young preschooler immediately labeled her stuttering as "sticky," because she felt the words were "getting stuck in my mouth." Other children identify with "bumps" on a country road and agree that "bumpy speech" would be a good label for their stuttering. Once the stuttering is out in the open and the child has words to describe it, directly addressing it in therapy is facilitated.

Some young children may not have developed the metalinguistic skills they need to think and talk about their speech. Although they are aware that speech is difficult at times, they may not be cognizant of individual instances of fluency breakdown. In this case, the clinician may want to choose a stuttering behavior that the child produces, model that behavior while at the same time minimizing struggle, and then label that behavior in words deemed appropriate for the child. The first author is working with a 3-year-old boy who used some struggled sound prolongations. During trial therapy, it was clear that this youngster was not overtly aware of fluency breakdown in his speech. The clinician, however, modeled some less tense prolongations and called them her "stretchy" speech. In that same session, the child soon consistently identified "stretchy" speech produced by the clinician and received tangible reinforcement for that identification. In the next session, the child began to point out the prolongations in his own speech in order to continue to play the "catch the stretchy speech" game. The use of imagery is beneficial in helping the child develop a mental picture of an abstract concept. Terms to describe stuttering that have been meaningful for children we have worked with include "bumpy," "sticky," "stretchy," and "jittery."

Once a meaningful label has been chosen, children are encouraged to listen for the "bumpy" speech and are rewarded for identifying it. We teach children how to play the speech "tag" game. When they hear "bumpy" speech, the children tag the clinician and receive points redeemable for a prize when the game is over. We pair the acknowledgment of an unpleasant behavior (stuttering) with the fun of playing "tag" and the anticipation of winning a prize. With no exceptions, this playful way of identifying stuttering has met with enthusiasm. Stuttering is no longer an overwhelming mystery, but something that now has boundaries.

The next goal in this approach to therapy is to teach the child how to change the quality of stuttering by substituting a less tense, more normal disfluency. We practice stuttering in a whisper, with a loud voice, with muscle tension, and when pretending to be asleep. When children are able to vary stuttering while producing disfluencies on purpose, we then show them how to stop after a moment of stuttering and say the word again changing the stuttering in some way. We methodically remove the layers of struggle behavior that have built up since the child started stuttering, beginning with the most advanced struggle behaviors. If children are prolonging sounds with pitch rise, we might show them how to prolong sounds in a more relaxed way without the rising pitch. If children are repeating parts of words numerous times, we will show them how to repeat syllables only one time. As the layers of struggle are removed, the child gradually replaces the abnormal disfluencies with normal fluency skills.

We begin this process of modifying stuttering by modeling the desired behavior in our own speech while playing with the child. Often children will imitate the less tense disfluency they hear without direct instruction. However, for other children it is necessary to show them how to substitute the more typical disfluency when a stuttering episode has occurred. Children are initially reinforced for any attempt to use a less tense disfluency. As skills develop, reinforcement is then reserved for modification attempts initiated by the child. When children discover that they have some control over speech fluency, the less tense disfluencies increase in number as the stuttering decreases.

It is sometimes helpful to teach the child to use normal disfluencies, even during fluent speech production. We call these normal disfluencies "easy bounces" and teach children how to use an easy, relaxed, whole word or phrase repetition at the beginning of sentences. These normal disfluencies then appear to take the place of stuttering.

Children may also benefit from learning the fluency enhancing skills modeled for them by the clinician.Learning to use a slower speech rate ("snail" speech versus "cheetah" speech) may be a useful treatment objective. Other children may use a louder voice in an effort to control fluency. They would benefit from practicing use of an "indoor" voice. The story of The Three Bears is sometimes helpful in this regard. We play the roles of each of the bears and discover that the Mama Bear used the best voice of all. When children still show signs of increased muscle tension during stuttering, we may teach them how to initiate phonation easily and maintain a low level of muscle tension while talking. Again, imagery is beneficial in teaching easy onset and light articulatory contacts to young children. We may talk about "sleepy time" speech and stretch out on the floor pretending we are just about ready to fall asleep. Then we practice talking in that more relaxed way. Other images we have found helpful include sliding into the base during a baseball game and gliding on ice with skates. We might also help the child use more continuous phonation by learning to "keep the motor going" while talking.

When the child has begun to use normal fluency most of the time, the clinician will slowly decrease use of a fluency enhancing interaction style. The child will be provided with opportunities to practice normal fluency skills while the clinician speaks more rapidly, asks more questions, occasionally interrupts, and increases the conversational pace. When the child is able to maintain normal fluency with increased demands in the clinic, practice is provided using these skills with family members at home, in the neighborhood with peers, and in the preschool classroom.

EVALUATION

Criteria for Dismissal

On discharge from therapy, we expect that the child's fluency levels will have approached normal levels. In addition, we expect that the child has shown resilience when fluency demands were increased in the clinic. Occasionally, children are discharged from direct therapy even when they have demonstrated some residual stuttering. However, these children have made increasing strides in mastering normal fluency, and their stuttering is not especially struggled. Their parents feel comfortable manipulating pertinent environmental variables. It is clear that, unless some unexpected factor were to occur, these children will continue to develop the skills needed to speak with normal fluency.

Environmental factors also play a role in determining a child's readiness for discharge from treatment. We hope that parents and teachers feel comfortable identifying and modifying environmental variables that are related to increases in stuttering. Families who are able to match the speech and interaction styles they use with their child's current developmental levels are able to provide a fluency enhancing environment. In this kind of environment, demands are minimized and capacities are allowed to flourish.

Prior to discharge, families are encouraged to develop a plan to deal with relapse, should it occur. Parents identify strategies they have found useful in shaping their child's fluency skills in the past. For example, parents may decide that if they notice the reemergence of stuttering they will reinitiate special interaction time, slow the pace of family activities, and more carefully monitor turn-taking. Before completing direct intervention, parents should feel comfortable in their knowledge of what to change should their child start stuttering and how to measure the effects of that change. The parents and clinician will also discuss when families should recontact the clinic should concerns about their child's fluency persist.

Follow-up Procedures

When children and their families have been discharged from direct intervention, they are asked to return to the clinic once every 3 months for the first 6 months and again 1 year from the discharge date. Periodic telephone contacts are made with the family during the second year postdischarge from therapy. During each contact, families are encouraged to call the clinic for a follow-up visit should concerns arise. Occasionally families return for short-term direct intervention if they feel they have been unable to make a difference in their child's fluency skills through environmental changes.

Results of Therapy

Between 1981 and 1989, 55 families received intervention through the Stuttering Prevention Center at Temple University in Philadelphia. Results of those interventions have been reported elsewhere (Starkweather et al., 1990). To summarize those results, 16 families participated in a limited stuttering treatment program; they were counseled via telephone contacts and provided with literature regarding stuttering prevention, and some participated in several family counseling sessions. All the children soon achieved normal fluency and those skills were maintained as measured by follow-up telephone contacts conducted for up to 2 years postinitial contact.

Of the remaining families, 39 were enrolled in direct treatment programs. Prior to completing their programs, 7 families withdrew, some moved away, and others decided the treatment program was not meeting their needs. During follow-up contacts, the children in 4 of these 7 families continued to stutter. Three of the 32 remaining families were in treatment at the time these results were reported. The children from the remaining 29 families successfully completed the intervention program and were discharged with normal fluency. All of these children continued to demonstrate normal fluency during follow-up visits and telephone contacts.

From 1993 through 1996, 15 families were treated in the southern New Hampshire area by the first author using the method described in this chapter. One family withdrew from the program prior to its completion and that child continues to stutter. The remaining 14 families were successfully discharged from treatment and then followed for fluency maintenance. All 14 children continue to use normal fluency as reported by their parents and as demonstrated in audiotapes of family interactions at home. The average duration of treatment was 14.5 sessions, including both family counseling and direct work with the child.

SUMMARY

In this chapter, we described a multiprocess early intervention program for young children who stutter and their families.

- We believe that stuttering develops when the child lacks the capacity to speak as fluently as the environment demands.
- The goals of the multiprocess intervention program are to reduce fluency demands while at the same time strengthening the child's fluency capacities.
- Parents and teachers receive accurate information about fluency and stuttering, learn to modify environmental factors directly related to the child's fluency, learn to communicate in ways that better match the child's current performance levels, and explore their feelings and attitudes related to their child's stuttering.

- Children learn to use a slow-normal speech rate; to reduce the struggle associated with stuttering, and to replace stuttering with normal fluency.

REFERENCES

Adams, M. R. (1990). The demands and capacities model I: Theoretical elaborations. *Journal of Fluency Disorders, 15,* 135–141.

Adams, M. R. (1992). Childhood stuttering under "positive" conditions. *American Journal of Speech-Language Pathology, 1,* 5–6.

Amster, B. (1984). *The development of speech rate in normal preschool children.* Unpublished doctoral dissertation, Temple University, Philadelphia.

Bell, H. (1986, November). *Topic changes as a predictor of stuttering in young children.* Poster session presented at the American Speech-Language-Hearing Convention, Detroit, MI.

Bernstein-Ratner, N. (1997). Leaving Las Vegas: Clinical odds and individual outcomes. *American Journal of Speech-Language Pathology, 6*(1), 29–33.

Culp, D. (1984). The preschool fluency development program: Assessment and treatment. In M. Peins (Ed.), *Contemporary approaches in stuttering therapy* (pp. 36–69). Boston: Little, Brown.

Curlee, R. F., & Yairi, E. (1997). Early intervention with early childhood stuttering: A critical examination of the data. *American Journal of Speech-Language Pathology, 6*(2), 8–18.

Gottwald, S. R., & Starkweather, C. W. (1995). Fluency intervention for preschoolers and their families in the public schools. *Language, Speech and Hearing Services in the Schools, 11,* 117–126.

Gregory, H., & Hill, D. (1980). Stuttering therapy for children. In W. Perkins (Ed.), *Stuttering disorders* (pp. 351–363). New York: Thieme-Stratton.

Guitar, B. (1998). *Stuttering: An integrated approach to its nature and treatment* (2nd ed.). Baltimore, MD: Williams & Wilkins.

Hill, D., & Campbell, J. (1987, November). *Systematic disfluency analysis.* Miniseminar presented at the American Speech-Language-Hearing Convention, New Orleans, LA.

Ingham, R. (1993). Current status of stuttering and behavior modification: II. Principles, issues, and practices. *Journal of Fluency Disorders, 18,* 57–80.

Kelly, E. M. (1994). Speech rates and turn-taking behaviors of children who stutter and their fathers. *Journal of Speech and Hearing Research, 37,* 1284–1294.

Kelly, E. M., & Conture, E. G. (1992). Speaking rates, response time latencies, and interrupting behaviors of young stutterers, non-stutterers, and their mothers. *Journal of Speech and Hearing Research, 35,* 1256–1267.

Kloth, S., Janssen, P., Kraaimaat, F., & Brutten, G. (1995). Speech-motor and linguistic skills of young stutterers prior to onset. *Journal of Fluency Disorders, 20*, 157–170.

Kowal, A., O'Connell, D. C., & Sabin, E. F. (1975). Development of temporal patterning and vocal hesitations in spontaneous narratives. *Journal of Psycholinguistic Research, 4*, 195–207.

Langlois, A., & Long, S. H. (1988). A model for teaching parents to facilitate fluent speech. *Journal of Fluency Disorders, 13*, 163–172.

Lincoln, M., & Onslow, M. (1997). Long-term outcomes of early intervention for stuttering. *American Journal of Speech-Language Pathology, 6*(1), 51–58.

Lincoln, M., Onslow, M., & Reed, V. (1997). Social validity of the treatment outcomes of an early intervention program for stuttering. *American Journal of Speech-Language Pathology, 6*(2), 77–84.

Manning, W. H. (1996). *Clinical decision making in the diagnosis and treatment of fluency disorders*. Albany, NY: Delmar Publishers.

Meyers, S. C. (1990). Verbal behaviors of preschool stutterers and conversational partners: Observing reciprocal relationships. *Journal of Speech and Hearing Disorders, 55*, 706–712.

Meyers, S. C. (1991). Interactions with pre-operational preschool stutterers: How will this influence therapy? In L. Rustin (Ed.), *Parents, families and the stuttering child* (pp. 40–58). Kibworth, UK: Far Communications.

Meyers, S. C., & Freeman, F. J. (1985a). Are mothers of stutterers different? An investigation of social-communicative interaction. *Journal of Fluency Disorders, 10*, 193–209.

Meyers, S. C., & Freeman, F. J. (1985b). Interruptions as a variable in stuttering and disfluency. *Journal of Speech and Hearing Research, 28*, 435–444.

Onslow, M., Andrews, C., & Lincoln, M. (1994). A control/experimental trial of an operant treatment for early stuttering. *Journal of Speech and Hearing Research, 37*, 1244–1259.

Riley, G. D. (1994). *Stuttering Severity Instrument for Children and Adults* (3rd ed.). Austin, TX: Pro-Ed.

Rustin, L. (1987). The treatment of childhood dysfluency through active parental involvement. In L. Rustin, H. Purser, & D. Rowley (Eds.), *Progress in the treatment of fluency disorders* (pp. 166–180). New York: Taylor & Francis.

Ryan, B. (1990, November). *Development of stuttering, a longitudinal study: Report 4*. Paper presented at the Annual Convention of the American Speech-Language-Hearing Association, Seattle, WA.

Shames, G., & Florence, S. (1980). *Stutter-free speech: A goal for therapy*. Columbus, OH: Charles Merrill.

Shine, R. (1984). Assessment and fluency training with the young stutterer. In M. Peins (Ed.), *Contemporary approaches in stuttering therapy* (pp. 173–216). Boston: Little, Brown.

Starkweather, C. W. (1987). *Fluency and stuttering*. Englewood Cliffs, NJ: Prentice-Hall.

Starkweather, C. W. (1997). Therapy for younger children. In R. Curlee & G. Siegel (Eds.), *Nature and treatment of stuttering: New directions* (2nd ed., pp. 257–279). Boston: Allyn & Bacon.

Starkweather, C. W., & Givens-Ackerman, J. (1997). *Stuttering*. Austin, TX: Pro-Ed.

Starkweather, C. W., & Gottwald, S. R. (1990). The demands and capacities model: II. Clinicial implications. *Journal of Fluency Disorders, 15,* 143–157.

Starkweather, C. W., & Gottwald, S. R. (1993). A pilot study of relations among specific measures obtained at intake and discharge in a program of prevention and early intervention for stuttering. *American Journal of Speech-Language Pathology, 2*(1), 51–58.

Starkweather, C. W., Gottwald, S. R., & Halfond, M. M. (1990). *Stuttering prevention: A clinical method.* Englewood Cliffs, NJ: Prentice-Hall.

Stocker, B. (1980). *The Stocker probe technique for diagnosis and treatment of stuttering in young children.* Tulsa, OK: Modern Education Corporation.

Wall, M. J., & Myers, F. L. (1995). *Clinical management of childhood stuttering* (2nd ed.). Austin, TX: Pro-Ed.

Watkins, R., & Yairi, E. (1997). Language production abilities of children whose stuttering persisted or recovered. *Journal of Speech, Language, and Hearing Research, 40,* 385–399.

Weiss, A. L., & Zebrowski, P. M. (1992). Disfluencies in the conversations of young children who stutter: Some answers about questions. *Journal of Speech and Hearing Research, 35,* 1230–1238.

Winslow, H., & Guitar, B. (1994). The effects of structured turn-taking on disfluencies: A case study. *Language, Speech and Hearing Services in the Schools, 25,* 251–257.

Yairi, E. H., & Ambrose, N. (1992). A longitudinal study of stuttering in children: A preliminary report. *Journal of Speech and Hearing Research, 35,* 755–760.

Yairi, E. H., Ambrose, N., Paden, E., & Throneburg, R. (1996). Predictive factors of persistence and recovery: Pathways of childhood stuttering. *Journal of Communication Disorders, 29,* 51–77.

Yaruss, J. S., & Conture, E. G. (1995). Mother and child speaking rates and utterance lengths in adjacent fluent utterances: Preliminary observations. *Journal of Fluency Disorders, 20,* 257–278.

Zebrowski, P. (1997). Assisting young children who stutter and their families: Defining the role of the speech-language pathologist. *American Journal of Speech-Language Pathology, 6*(2), 19–28.

4

Developmental Intervention: Differential Strategies

HUGO H. GREGORY

INTRODUCTION

When parents express concern that their child is "stuttering" or "beginning to stutter," we do an evaluation to determine (a) whether there should or should not be concern about the child's speech, and (b) if there is concern, what child developmental or environmental factors should be focused on to either prevent the development of stuttering or to "stem the tide" of a developing problem. The process, called "differential evaluation," leads to the adoption of different therapeutic strategies, taking into consideration the needs of each child and family. I speak of this as "developmental intervention" because we are taking action to influence a child's speech and language during a period of rapid development and at a time when growth and development favor the child becoming more fluent (Gregory & Hill, 1980, 1993, 1998). Before describing specific procedures of differential evaluation—differential therapy, a brief historical review of experiences in early intervention at Northwestern University is given to show the reader how this early intervention activity evolved.

Historical Perspective

For all children with speech and language problems who come to the Northwestern Speech and Language Clinic, there is a long tradition of doing a broad evaluation covering many aspects of children's development and their environment. Thereafter, as has been true at most clinics, initial decisions about therapy have been based on evaluation findings. When I was a graduate student at Northwestern during the 1950s, a program of early intervention was initiated with children found to be beginning to stutter, in which they were seen for individual and group therapy and parents were counseled. During my early years on the Northwestern faculty, beginning in 1962, Van Riper's desensitization method (Van Riper, 1954) was the basis for early intervention, always taking into consideration concomitant problems such as those of articulation or language and issues related to family interaction. In 1966, a guidebook for parents and therapists dealing with these children was prepared (Walvoord & Hall, 1966).

Influenced by Bandura's research on observational learning, modeling, and reinforcement (Bandura, 1969), Gregory (1973), and Hill and Gregory (1975) found that, in many cases, the process of normalizing fluency in preschool children was facilitated by reinforcing children for imitating a clinician's more easy relaxed speech in a play atmosphere. Desensitization, like Van Riper's method (Van Riper, 1954), was used as judged to be appropriate after speech responses began to change (Gregory & Hill, 1980, 1993). In addition, in about 1975 we began to utilize observational learning to assist parents in making changes in their communicative and interpersonal behaviors that, based on a case history and a parent-child interaction analysis, were observed to be related to the child's increased disfluency and stuttering. Parents first observe how the clinician interacts with the child, for example, speaking in a more relaxed and phrased manner. They may observe the way in which the clinician allows more pause time after the child talks and before the adult speaks again. This is labeled as "delaying your response." Parents then practice these behaviors in a therapy session. Later, these behaviors are practiced at home. Parents have responded positively to this modeling approach, reporting that they gained confidence in their ability to change by first knowing more precisely what they should do. They have also expressed appreciation for the feedback given as they attempted to modify their behavior. In this way, widely used cognitive-verbal interaction approaches to counseling have been combined with more cognitive-behavior change procedures. We have come to believe that a key element in the success of intervention is a positive relationship between the parents and the clinician, as well as between the clinician and the child.

This chapter describes our present approach to preschool intervention, revealing how I have profited from my collaboration for 25 years with Diane Hill, who has specialized in early intervention and is in every way a master clinician, and from work with my wife, Carolyn, who has had a special impact on my understanding of the emotional aspects of children's speech problems and parent counseling.

THE PROGRAM

Differential Evaluation

In the last 25 years, coinciding with my experience, several contributors, among them Riley and Riley (1979, 1983), Starkweather, Gottwald, and Halfond (1990), and Wall and Meyers (1995), have advocated systems for evaluation based on the belief that it is important to recognize individual differences from child to child. Of course, Van Riper's pioneering work influenced all of us (Van Riper, 1973).

The diagram in Figure 4–1 is an overview of the decisions made in differential evaluation—differential treatment (Gregory & Hill, 1993, 1998). In this system, the level of initial evaluation is determined by information received from the parents, often by a telephone call stating their concern. A fluency screening evaluation is carried out if parents describe a pattern of speech disruption that seems typical of children at the child's age or if stuttering has been of concern for less than 6 months and no concern is expressed about other aspects of speech and language development. This evaluation consists of (a) a brief case history of speech, language, and fluency development; (b) an analysis of fluency as noted in monologue, play, play with pressure, and parent-child interaction; (c) an analysis of parent-child interactive behaviors, such as rapid turn-taking; and (d) a brief assessment of other aspects of speech and language and a screening of hearing. Decisions following this evaluation may result in utilizing Treatment Strategy I (Preventive Parent Counseling) or Strategy II (Prescriptive Parent Counseling and Limited Involvement of the Child) or in scheduling an in-depth speech and language evaluation. An in-depth evaluation includes all of the widely used diagnostic procedures and a more detailed assessment of the four areas mentioned earlier. Such an evaluation is also done if the initial contact indicates that stuttering has been a concern for 6 months or longer or if there is concern about other aspects

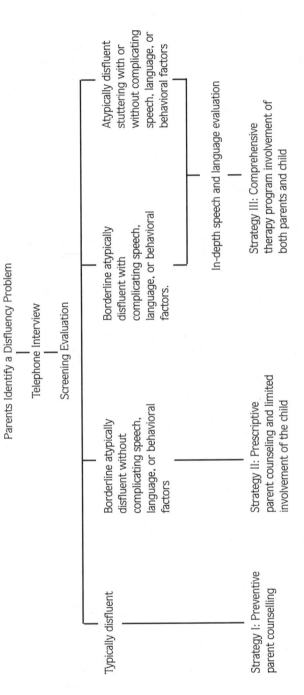

Figure 4-1. Overview of differential evaluation in therapy. (From "Stuttering Therapy for Children, by H. H. Gregory and D. Hill, 1984. p. 78. In W. Perkins (Ed.), *Stuttering Disorders*. New York: Thieme-Stratton, Inc. Reprinted with permission.)

of the child's speech and language development. Ordinarily, an in-depth speech and language evaluation leads to the child's and parents' involvement in Treatment Strategy III (Comprehensive Therapy Program; Involvement of Both Parents and Child).[1]

Differential Treatment Strategies

In making clinical judgments about a child's fluency and in making decisions with parents about intervention, we have found it helpful to think about disfluency in children's speech along a continuum from "More Usual" at one end to "More Unusual" at the other. In several publications beginning with Gregory and Hill (1980) and in revisions of this continuum over the years (Gregory & Hill, 1993, 1998), research information and clinical observations have been summarized to provide a rationale for this continuum.

More Typical Disfluencies on the Continuum Are in Order of Expected Frequency:

Hesitations (silent pauses), interjections of sounds, syllables, or words, revisions of phrases or sentences, phrase repetitions, one-syllable word repetitions (two or fewer repetitions per instance, even stress, no noticeable tension), part-word repetitions (two or fewer repetitions per instance, even stress, no noticeable tension).

Atypical Disfluencies-Stuttering in Order of Tension Involved and Amount of Disruption of Speech Flow:

One-syllable word repetitions (three or more repetitions per instance or uneven stress), part-word syllable repetitions (three or more repetitions per instance or uneven stress), sound repetitions, prolongations, blocks, tremor of lips or jaw or vocal tension.

Using disfluency data from the *Systematic Disfluency Analysis*, a method for identifying and quantifying a full range of disfluencies (Campbell & Hill, 1987), and employing the *Continuum of Disfluency Behavior* described above in summary form, we classify patterns into the following diagnostic categories (Gregory & Hill, 1993, 1998):

[1] Differential evaluation, including an analysis of fluency, assessment of environmental factors, and an evaluation of other speech, language, and behavioral factors, is described in Gregory and Hill (1993, 1998).

- **Typically disfluent:** Less than 10% typical disfluency and less than 2% atypical disfluency (stuttering)
- **Borderline atypically disfluent:** 10% or more typical disfluency and/or 2 to 3% atypical disfluency
- **Atypically disfluent/stuttering:** 3% or more atypical disfluency and/or 10% or more total disfluency.

We are well aware of the variability of stuttering! Therefore, it is important to sample fluency across several speaking situations, as mentioned previously in describing the screening evaluation. The reader will recognize that monologue, play, play with pressure, and parent-children interaction or such situations as storytelling reflect the effects of different communication variables. How these fluency criteria and other information from a case history and clinical observation and testing are used in determining initial intervention decisions is described in the next section. Concise descriptions of three treatment strategies follow. All clinicians integrate what we share about our experience into their own practices, and it is expected that readers will do so.

Treatment Strategy I: Preventive Parent Counseling

Even when my judgment following a screening evaluation is that parents are concerned about disfluency that seems to be within normal limits, I have found it appropriate to do some short-term parent counseling. This is especially important if the parents believe that what we have observed may not be characteristic, that the child does show more disruption of fluency than revealed during the screening. It may also be necessary if parents appear especially sensitive about disfluency in a child's speech, for example, displaying an awareness associated with a father who has a history of stuttering. Such counseling proceeds along the following lines:

1. I listen to the parents' descriptions of their observations and concerns with a genuine desire to understand. I reward them for sharing their thoughts and feelings by saying such things as, "Telling me about this is very helpful in understanding your child's speech and your child's feelings about talking at the present time."
2. I describe speech development, including information about the occurrence of disfluency in children's speech, perhaps using the continuum as a frame of reference. We help parents to understand the basis for our judgment that their child's disfluency at the present time

is typical for his or her age. This feedback is conducted in a relaxed way, creating an atmosphere in which parents feel unhurried and comfortable to question what we are saying.

3. I discuss some communicative and interpersonal situations that in my experience have been related to increased disfluency in children. It is best to build on some situation that parents mention, such as conversation at meal time. I reinforce some appropriate and positive behaviors on the parents' part before turning attention to some behaviors that could interrupt fluency development. For example, if the mother says that she tries to be especially calm when she sees that her child is very excited, this can be reinforced. If the father says that everyone interrupts each other at the dinner table, that can be discussed with reference to turn-taking and how to manage it. For example, I usually tell parents that they should first model better turn-taking when talking to each other, and when they interrupt, say "Excuse me." Parents have been interested in my explanation of improving conversational skills by commenting more on what each is saying, rather than questioning so much!

4. The concept of time pressure in communication is discussed. I present time pressure as a natural part of communication and give concrete examples of how disfluency is increased by adults and children attempting to compete in conversations. I explain that children, during their preschool years when speech and language are developing, need more time to think about what they want to say and to formulate language. It can be related to turn-taking. I recommend that parents learn to pause "to the count of two in your mind" before they begin to talk after a child has finished an utterance.

5. In terms of child rearing in general, parents find it helpful to understand the demand/support ratio as it was described by Sheehan (1970, 1979) in his writing about childhood stuttering. If parents are giving children considerable support by spending time with them and reinforcing them (praising) for desirable behavior, they then are in a better position to make certain demands. Support should always outweigh demands. I mention this because I believe that interpersonal stress

is sometimes a factor contributing to stuttering problems. Parents have said that this discussion has helped them understand how to interact with their child in a more positive manner.

6. I reinforce information given by having parents read *If Your Child Stutters: A Guide for Parents* (Ainsworth & Gruss, 1981) and *Stuttering and Your Child: Questions and Answers* (Conture & Fraser, 1989), distributed by the Stuttering Foundation of America.

One or two counseling sessions are usually sufficient to help parents feel more secure about a child's speech. Several monthly telephone contacts are ordinarily planned to confirm the parents' satisfaction or to recognize a continuing need, either for parent counseling or another evaluation.

Treatment Strategy II: Prescriptive Parent Counseling, Brief Therapy With the Child

If a child is judged to be borderline atypically disfluent, even if there are no concomitant articulation, language, or behavioral problems that may be complicating the problem, the strategy of seeing both the child and the parents for brief therapy, usually four to six sessions, is recommended. In counseling parents, the general procedure of being a careful, interested listener, of gradually providing information about speech and language development, and of describing our knowledge about the characteristics of children's disfluency and stuttering are, in general, the same as those discussed under Strategy I. The following procedures are specific to Strategy II:

1. Based on observations made and information gained in the screening evaluation, feedback is given to the parents about judgments of the child's disfluency and other speech and language skills. The parents are trained to identify the different types of repetitious disfluencies (i.e., sound, syllable, and word repetition) and nonrepetitious disfluencies (i.e., pauses, interjections, and revisions) through the use of videotaped examples. They are also shown how tension can enter into a child's speech production to make repetitions faster, prolongations longer, and result in repetitions becoming prolongations, blocks, tremors, and so on.

2. Parents are given instruction in charting instances of disfluency during a day, and these charts are brought to counseling sessions for discussion. The following chart (see Table 4–1) from Gregory and Hill (1993) illustrates the information recorded by a parent and reported to the clinician, perhaps at a counseling session with a group of parents. These charts lead not only to analyses of situations in which disfluency occurred, associated circumstances, and an evaluation of parents' reactions, but also to a discussion of parent-child interactions in general, such as discipline and preparing for an exciting experience like a party or holiday.

3. The child is seen for 30- to 50-minute sessions twice a week The child and the clinician are involved in activities that promote fluency, and as soon as possible a parent joins in the session. In clinics where there is an observation room, the parent may watch from there at first, with another clinician to explain what is occurring. I model an easy, relaxed, somewhat slower speaking manner with an emphasis on pausing between phrases, being a responsive listener as the child talks, and showing the child how we take turns—adults don't interrupt and neither does the child. The clinician reads stories or engages the child in a game, talking in an easy-relaxed manner. It has always been as-

Table 4–1. Chart of disfluent episodes.

Person	Message	Type of Disfluency	Child Awareness	Listener Reaction	Fluency Disruptors
Mother talkng on phone	Child interrupted his mother and wanted to get her attention	Irregular rhythm on syllable repetitions in the first word of the sentence	Overall tense but not aware of disfluencies	Mother said she would talk as soon as she finished	Getting listener attention, not tolerant of delay

Source: From "Differential Evaluation—Differential Therapy for Stuttering Children," by H. Gregory and D. Hill, 1993, p. 32. In *Stuttering and Related Disorders*, R. Curlee (Ed.). New York: Thieme Medical Publishers. Reprinted with permission.

tonishing to me how rapidly many of these children, especially those 2 and 3 years of age, modify their speech in response to a more relaxed model. In some cases, the clinician may give an instruction, "Make your speech easy like mine." During the second or third session, after receiving some individual instruction, a parent is asked to modify her or his speech when talking with the child in the therapy session. As soon as possible, home assignments are given.

4. A key to successful work during the last 20 years has been that parents have practiced and learned improved interactive behaviors, both in communication and behavior in general. For example, parents have profited from seeing how the clinician plays calmly with the child, models turn-taking, or comments on what the child says and reduces the number of questions. It is pointed out how commenting on what the child says signals that the parent is interested and listening and, at the same time, nourishes the child's self-esteem. Modeling is a powerful approach (Bandura, 1969; Gregory, 1973) and one easily understood by clinicians and by parents. Most parents want to learn to respond appropriately, and once they get into the process of change, it is usually rewarding to them. Also, it is good for the children to know that their parents are learning, too.

Four to eight weekly sessions are usually sufficient to accomplish normal fluency in the child and for the parents to believe that they understand the variables that require monitoring. Furthermore, the parents are showing an ability to make appropriate changes; for example, when the child shows a little more stuttering, it is now a signal to the parents to be more relaxed in their manner, to increase pause time while speaking, and to pause between the time the child stops talking and they begin. Plans are made for follow-up telephone contacts and post-treatment observations at the clinic, as needed. If, at any time, parents have concerns about increased disfluency, we advise them by telephone to assist problem solving or, if indicated, see the family.

Treatment Strategy III: Comprehensive Therapy Program

As indicated in Figure 4–1, this treatment plan is designed for the child who is borderline atypically disfluent with complicating speech, language, or behavioral problems and also the atypically disfluent child (demonstrating more definite stuttering behaviors) in whom we may or may not have found contributing speech, language, or behavioral factors. Often, parents report concern about speech disfluencies that have persisted for more than 6 months and sometimes longer than a year, with decreasing cyclic variation. In my experience, greater cyclic variation indicates a better prognosis. Most often these children are 3 or 4 years of age. These children are seen two to four times a week for 30- to 50-minute sessions, and the parents should be counseled weekly. The child may be included in a children's group as change occurs, as the children can model for each other.

Most of what has been said about parent counseling in discussing Strategies I and II, aimed toward reducing communicative and interpersonal stress, is true for Strategy III. In brief, the clinician should be an understanding, interested listener, who is careful to comprehend the unique concerns of the parents and their family situation. Parents are usually relieved to know that the clinician is a person who can be of assistance. The clinician describes the development of speech with an emphasis on the development of fluency and the occurrence of disfluencies, discusses time pressure in communication, demands placed on the child compared to support, and other factors that may contribute to increased disfluency and stuttering. As described in Strategy II, the parents are taught to recognize different types of disfluency and to chart environmental situations that are associated with increases and decreases in disfluency. The following principles and procedures are more specific to Strategy III.

Differential Treatment.   The following two case illustrations show how treatment is based on the results of an evaluation that determines the nature of the problem, focusing on both child developmental factors and environmental factors believed to be contributing to the problem:

Brad, age 3 years, 7 months

Onset: Parents first noticed "sound repetition" at 2 years, 6 months.

Speech analysis: Evaluation revealed moderately severe stuttering, a high frequency of sound and syllable repetitions, sound prolongations, and laryngeal tension (loud, hard, glottal attacks). There was considerable situational variation in frequency of disfluency.

Developmental factors: Language, articulation, hearing, and motor skills (including oral motor) were within normal limits.

Environmental factors: Parent-child interaction revealed that mother spoke with a rapid rate and used demanding questions frequently. At times, two or three consecutive questions were asked without allowing time for Brad to respond. Mother interrupted Brad's comments. Parent and child appeared to have a positive emotional relationship, and there were no signs of significant parent-child conflict.

Warren, age 4 years

Onset: Around his third birthday, parents were concerned about stuttering that included tense repetitions of sounds and syllables.

Speech analysis: Repetitions of sounds, syllables, and one-syllable words at the beginning of a phrase. Repetitions characterized by relatively even rhythm. Occasionally, there were short breaths between repetitions. There were only a few prolongations. Stuttering classified as mild. He was able to imitate a model of easy, relaxed speech readily and some immediate carryover was noted.

Developmental factors: All developmental milestones, including speech and language, essentially normal. No significant medical problems. Speech and language abilities within normal range at present. Psychological evaluation resulted in an IQ of 105, which the psychologist thought was probably lower than his actual operating level since several failures on tasks represented "resistance to the task and attention problems." Index of social maturity 1 year below age level. Psychologist concluded that child was overanxious and insecure emotionally.

Environmental factors: Mother described Warren as loving, sensitive, and intelligent. She also said that he was anxious, aggressive, and sometimes stubborn, "a boy who requires a great deal of discipline." Parents consulted a pediatrician a few months earlier about temper tantrums. Mother suspects that "he acts out to get attention." During the last year he has been in a nursery school where no behavior problems have been observed.

With Brad, the emphasis was on counseling the parents about communicative stress (the way in which parents and others talked to the child), modeling improved interactive behaviors such as turn-taking, and rewarding the parents for making changes in their behavior. In working with Brad, the clinician modeled a more easy, slightly slower, relaxed speech pattern, going from shorter to longer utterances and from less meaningful to more meaningful (naming, descriptions, interpretations). The parents were taught to modify their speech rate and to pause more frequently. The core period of therapy was 6 months with follow-up to make sure normal fluency was stabilized.

With Warren, emotional-social development and parent-child relationships were the main concerns. Parents and child were seen for a 3-month period during which the psychological evaluation (mentioned above) was done. Warren responded well to the clinician's model of easy relaxed speech. The mother and father were taught general bodily relaxation procedures and were able to adopt a slower, more relaxed speaking rate. The parents followed the clinician's model in learning to set limits on Warren's behavior and to reinforce his behavior when he was more cooperative and less demanding. However, when the mother entered the therapy room, Warren often would cling to her and become more disfluent. Based on observations in the clinic and the psychological evaluation, Warren and the parents were referred for family-oriented psychotherapy as speech therapy continued. Four months later, Warren and family were dismissed from both therapies and his speech was normal. In psychotherapy, it was said that he had worked through his insecurities; clinging to the mother was much less than before. The mother gained insight into the way in which it was possible that her son's aggressive and clinging behaviors were a way of controlling her. But, of course, Warren also needed to feel more self-confident, and the positive reinforcement and boosting of his self-esteem received in both therapies helped.

These two brief examples illustrate how differential evaluation leads to different treatment approaches and how each child and family are unique. Topics discussed next describe in greater detail some of the procedures referred to in these examples.

Facilitating the Child's Fluency.   An analysis of the literature on early intervention indicates a trend during the last 25 years toward the increased use of fluency enhancing procedures, ranging in terms of direct speech modification from Ryan's gradual increase in length and complexity (GILCU; Ryan, 1974, 1979), to Costello-

Ingham's extended length of fluent utterances (ELU; Costello, 1984; Costello-Ingham, 1993), to the modeling of a slightly slower, more easy relaxed speech pattern by Gregory and Hill (1980, 1993, 1998), to a soft vocal production by Shine (1984), to what appears to be the most direct procedure, that of Cooper and Cooper (1985) using fluency enhancing gestures (slow speech, easy speech, deep breath, loudness variation, smooth speech and stress variations). Gregory (1986) recommended facilitating normal fluency by focusing on the minimal number of parameters necessary. The clinician can always decide to increase the number of parameters of speech attended to, depending on the vocal tract dynamics of the child's stuttering and what is effective (Adams, 1984). Most recently, Onslow, Andrews, and Lincoln's technique (1994) of asking a child to repeat a stuttered utterance (verbal response-contingent punishment) and praising stutter-free speech is an approach to enhancing fluency by contingency management only. In my practice, I have not employed direct fluency enhancing procedures until it has been found that modifying psychosocial factors does not produce the desired speech improvement.

Gregory and Hill (1980, 1993, 1998) have employed a modeling procedure in which the child observes first the clinician and then the mother and father speak in a way that we call "slower more easy relaxed speech." Gregory and Hill (1998, p. 32) stated:

> Because children of 2 to 5 years of age are still developing perceptual, speech motor skills, the clinician's model must be quite obvious at first. Speech rate is slow and smooth. . . . Rate of speech is normalized as instruction in easy relaxed speech moves from words to phrases and longer utterances, and as these modifications become more stable in the child's speech.

The authors described the way in which easy relaxed speech is stabilized by practice moving through hierarchies relating not only to length of utterance, but also to increased propositionality (imitation, stereotyped response, short description, longer description, short conversation, longer conversation, etc.) and situational difficulty (on the floor, standing, walking, talking to another child, talking to parent, etc.). One of the most important functions of the clinician is to arrange for appropriately graduated steps of practice.

As a child's fluency stabilizes, specialized desensitization procedures, based on Van Riper's work (Van Riper, 1954), are applied as it seems appropriate. Based on an analysis of parent-child interactions and observations of the child during therapy, the clinician constructs a hierarchy of factors that disrupt the child's fluency. At first, disrupters of lower strength are applied and then gradually, as the child's fluency remains stable when these stimuli are introduced, disrupters higher in the hierarchy are introduced in a systematic manner. These procedures increase the child's tolerance of factors that once disrupted fluency and should be done only by the clinician, not by the parents (Gregory & Hill, 1993, 1998).

Attending to Concomitant Problems.   Some children seen for a fluency problem may also have an articulation, language, or behavior problem. Nippold (1990) reviewed and commented on studies related to these concomitant problems, and Ratner (1995) offered guidelines for the assessment and treatment of these related impairments. In working on fluency, we have mentioned that procedures to facilitate fluency are carried out in the context of language activities (e.g., working from shorter to longer utterances and from utterances involving less complex syntax to ones that are more complex). Thus, various syntactic structures can be incorporated as we improve fluency. In addition, once a child is responding positively in therapy, ordinarily with improved fluency, articulation problems can be managed with a relaxed, developmental approach. Word finding can be improved by associating the names of objects and pictures in terms of semantic attributes such as function, size, shape, color, and taste and by creating situations in which these words are used by the child. Parents are advised to provide word choices, perhaps saying, "Were you thinking of a banana, an apple, or an orange?" All of these articulation and language activities must be monitored to make sure that the child is not experiencing pressure that could increase stuttering.

If a child seems shy and tends to be withdrawn, the clinician may need to use more of a play therapy approach before beginning the fluency enhancing strategies described above. If the child is difficult to structure and tends to be recalcitrant, some time may be devoted to establishing limits and building rapport by reinforcing what the child does well. Again, we are reminded that we respond to each child in terms of his or her individual characteristics. Speech intervention always involves problem solving.

Generalization and Transfer.   With reference to the treatment strategies for early developmental stages and the involvement of parents in the process, generalization should occur readily, and our experience has been that this is usually the case. What Griffiths and Craighead (1972) term "intratherapy generalisation" takes place as a child learns to modify speech, first in small units such as words and phrases, then in phrases and sentences. At first, in terms of communicative responsibility, the response may be an imitated naming response, then naming without a model, then naming one object or picture when the model is given on another one, and so on. "Extratherapy generalisation" refers to the child generalizing change from individual therapy to a group session with other children or to a different listener (e.g., the mother) in the therapy setting. As described earlier, at first the parents observe the clinician and the child and follow the clinician's model. In the usual progression, the parents are given assignments to do at home what they have done at the clinic. Thus, both parents and child are experiencing generalization and transfer (Gregory, 1984). Again, we are joining with the parents to shape the developmental process! Follow-up rechecks should be done by telephone and the child should be brought in for a recheck whenever the parents express a need for reassurance.

EVALUATION

In prescriptive parent counseling, which is seen as preventive, we are nearly 100% successful after four to six sessions, ordinarily over a period of 2 to 4 weeks. Success is defined as the removal of parental concern and, in addition, the parents having learned enough to respond appropriately to the child's communication. This has been true at the Northwestern Speech Clinic and in a private practice. In only a few cases do parents of children for whom prescriptive parent counseling was thought to be appropriate show concern that requires further intervention.

In the comprehensive therapy program, successful intervention may take 6 to 12 months. Approximately 5% of these children and their parents have problems that are persistent and require longer term follow-up, which may also require referral for family counseling or psychoeducational evaluation. For example, one mother appeared very insecure about her ability to cope with the demands of her family, including making changes in her communicative behavior. A referral for family counseling was made. Some parents do not accept a recommendation for referral and some do not follow up on making communicative changes in the home beyond a short term. We stay in touch with parents and encourage them to let us help as appropriate and desired. Sometimes in responding to our inquiry parents will say that all is well, and sometimes they say, "I was just thinking about calling you. We have a few questions." Our experience at Northwestern and in a private practice agrees with that of most contributors (e.g., Conture, 1990; Meyers & Woodford, 1992; Riley & Riley, 1983; Starkweather et al., 1990) in finding that early intervention (especially during the first year after onset) is highly successful in normalizing speech development and preventing stuttering (Gregory & Hill, 1993, 1998).

Parents have always been told that "we have development on our side," and that, "we are joining with you to, hopefully, insure the normal development of speech for your child." Thus we have not fooled ourselves, or the parents, about development or "spontaneous recovery" playing a role in the progress observed. Again, this is why the designation "developmental intervention" is used.

SUMMARY

- A differential evaluation procedure is used in determining whether or not there should be concern about a child's speech and, if there is concern, what child developmental or environmental factors appear to be contributing to the problem.
- Considering the nature and degree of disfluency in a child's speech and the existence of complicating speech, language, and behavioral factors results in using one of three treatment strategies: Preventive Parent Counseling, Prescriptive Parent Counseling, or a Comprehensive Therapy Program.
- Transfer of improved fluency and follow-up of progress are important considerations.
- In Prescriptive Parent Counseling, which is seen as preventive, we are nearly 100% successful after four to six sessions,
- In the Comprehensive Therapy Program, successful intervention may take 6 to 12 months, and approximately 5% of these children and their parents have problems that are persistent and require longer term follow-up.

REFERENCES

Adams, M. (1984). The young stutterer: Diagnosis, treatment and assessment of progress. In W. Perkins (Ed.), *Stuttering disorders: Current therapy of communication disorders* (pp. 41–56). New York: Thieme-Stratton.

Ainsworth, S., & Gruss, J. (Eds.). (1981). *If your child stutters: A guide for parents* (Publ. No. 11). Memphis, TN: Stuttering Foundation of America.

Bandura, A. (1969). *Principles of behavior modification.* New York: Holt, Rinehart and Winston.

Campbell, J., & Hill, D. (1987). *Systematic disfluency analysis.* Unpublished manuscript.

Conture, E. (1990). *Stuttering.* Englewood Cliffs, NJ: Prentice-Hall.

Conture, E., & Fraser, J. (1989). *Stuttering and your child: Questions and answers* (Publ. No. 22). Memphis, TN: Stuttering Foundation of America.

Cooper, E., & Cooper, C. (1985). *Cooper personalised fluency control therapy—revised.* Allen, TX: DLM Teaching Resources.

Costello, J. (1984). Treatment of the young chronic stutterer: Managing fluency. In R. Curlee & W. Perkins (Eds.), *The nature and treatment of stuttering: New directions* (pp. 375–396). San Diego, CA: College-Hill Press.

Costello-Ingham, J. (1993). Behavioral treatment of stuttering children. In R. Curlee (Ed.), *Stuttering and other disorders of fluency* (pp. 68–100). New York: Thieme Medical Publishers.

Gregory, H. (1973). Modeling procedures in the treatment of elementary school age children who stutter. *Journal of Fluency Disorders, 1,* 58–63.

Gregory, H. (1984). Prevention of stuttering: Management of early stages. In R. Curlee & W. Perkins (Eds.), *Nature and treatment of stuttering: New directions* (pp. 335–356). San Diego, CA: College-Hill Press.

Gregory, H. (1986). *Stuttering: Differential evaluation and therapy.* Austin, TX: Pro-Ed.

Gregory, H., & Hill, D. (1980). Stuttering therapy for children. In W. Perkins (Ed.), *Strategies in stuttering therapy* (pp. 351–364). New York: Thieme-Stratton.

Gregory, H., & Hill, D. (1993). Differential evaluation-differential therapy for stuttering children. In R. Curlee (Ed.), *Stuttering and related disorders of fluency* (pp. 23–44). New York: Thieme Medical Publishers.

Gregory, H., & Hill, D. (1998). Differential evaluation—differential therapy for stuttering children. In R. Curlee (Ed.), *Stuttering and related disorders of fluency* (2nd ed., pp. 22–42). New York: Thieme Medical Publishers.

Griffiths, H., & Craighead, W. (1972). Generalization in operant speech therapy for misarticulation. *Journal of Speech and Hearing Disorders, 37,* 485–495.

Hill, D., & Gregory, H. (1975, March). *Modeling speech change in children who stutter.* Paper presented at the annual conference of the Illinois Speech and Hearing Association, Chicago, IL.

Meyers, S., & Woodford, L. (1992). *The fluency development system for young children*. Buffalo, NY: United Educational Services.

Nippold, M. (1990). Concomitant speech and language disorders in stuttering children: A critique of the literature. *Journal of Speech and Hearing Disorders, 55*, 51–60.

Onslow, M., Andrews, C., & Lincoln, M. (1994). A control/experimental trial of an operant treatment for early stuttering. *Journal of Speech and Hearing Research, 37*, 1244–1259.

Ratner, N. (1995). Treating the child who stutters with concomitant language or phonological impairment. *Language, Speech and Hearing Services in Schools, 26*, 180–186.

Riley, G., & Riley, J. (1979). A component model for diagnosing and treating children who stutter. *Journal of Fluency Disorders, 4*, 279–293.

Riley, G., & Riley, J. (1983). Evaluation as a basis for intervention. In D. Prins & R. Ingham (Eds), *Treatment of stuttering in early childhood* (pp. 43–67). San Diego, CA: College-Hill Press.

Ryan, B. (1974). *Programmed therapy for stuttering in children and adults*. Springfleld, IL: Charles C. Thomas.

Ryan, B. (1979). Stuttering therapy in a framework of operant conditioning and programmed learning. In H. Gregory (Ed.), *Controversies about stuttering therapy* (pp. 129–176). Austin, TX: Pro-Ed.

Sheehan, J. (1970). Role therapy. In J. Sheehan (Ed.), *Stuttering: Research and therapy* (pp. 260–311). New York: Harper and Row.

Sheehan, J. (1979). Current issues on stuttering and recovery. In H. Gregory (Ed.), *Controversies about stuttering therapy* (pp. 175–208). Baltimore: University Park Press.

Shine, R. (1984). Direct management of the beginning stutterer. In W. Perkins (Ed.), *Strategies in stuttering therapy* (pp. 339–350). New York: Thieme-Stratton.

Starkweather, C., Gottwald, S., & Halfond, M. (1990). *Stuttering prevention: A clinical method*. Englewood Cliffs, NJ: Prentice–Hall.

Van Riper, C. (1954). *Speech correction: Principles and methods*. Englewood Cliffs, NJ: Prentice-Hall.

Van Riper, C. (1973). *The treatment of stuttering*. Englewood Cliffs, NJ: Prentice-Hall.

Wall, M., & Myers, F. (1995). *Clinical management of childhood stuttering*. Austin, TX: Pro-Ed.

Walvoord, B., & Hall, N. (1966). *The prevention of stuttering*. Evanston, IL: Junior League of Evanston.

5

The Lidcombe Program

MICHELLE LINCOLN
ELISABETH HARRISON

INTRODUCTION

The Lidcombe Program is an early intervention for stuttering that originated in Sydney, Australia. The program is a result of collaboration between speech-language pathologists from the Stuttering Unit at Bankstown Health Service and researchers from the School of Communication Sciences and Disorders and the Australian Stuttering Research Centre at the University of Sydney. This collaboration began in the mid-1980s, when these speech-language pathologists and researchers worked in Lidcombe, a suburb in western Sydney. The program's name was chosen to reflect that geographical context. The Stuttering Unit and the Communication Disorders Treatment and Research Clinic at the University of Sydney are now situated in multicultural, medium to low socioeconomic level suburbs of Sydney, namely Bankstown and Lidcombe.

The chapter begins with a brief summary of the development of the Lidcombe Program. An overview of the program follows, and the chapter concludes with a summary of research projects in progress, and outcomes to date.

Development of the Lidcombe Program

The Lidcombe Program has its foundations in research that investigated the Operant properties of stuttering. The program emerged directly from the work of others who applied behavioral principles to the treatment of stuttering in adults and children (see Ingham [1984] for a summary). Behavioral therapies based on operant methodology target the signs of stuttering, repetitions, prolongations, and blocks, rather than the cause of stuttering.

Influences of Behavior Therapy on Preschool Treatments for Stuttering

While much research effort was devoted to exploring the effect of response-contingent stimulation on the speech of adult, adolescent, and school-age people who stutter, it was not until 1972 that the effect of response-contingent stimulation on the speech of preschool children was reported. In a landmark study with two preschool children, Martin, Kuhl, and Haroldson (1972) investigated the effect of time-out from speaking contingent on stutters. During weekly individual treatment sessions the children conversed with a puppet that was enclosed in an illuminated glass case. Contingent on stuttering, the puppet stopped talking and illumination ceased. After 10 seconds the case was reilluminated and the interaction continued. Immediate stuttering reductions occurred and generalized in the laboratory. Reed and Godden (1977) told two preschool children to slow down contingent on stutters. This technique eliminated stuttering; however, it is unclear whether stuttering was reduced because of the application of contingencies or because the children reduced their speech rate. Despite the encouraging results of these studies, other operant treatments for preschool stuttering children were not reported until the 1990s.

In 1990 Onslow, Costa, and Rue published a preliminary report of a parent-administered, response-contingent treatment program for stuttering preschool children. Onslow, Andrews, and Lincoln (1994) used the same treatment program with 13 preschool children who stuttered. In further publications the treatment program described by Onslow et al. (1990, 1994) was referred to as the Lidcombe Program. These later studies suggested that operant methodology may be effective with people of all ages who stutter.

THE PROGRAM

Client Population

The Lidcombe Program was developed for preschool-age children who stutter, that is, children under 5 years of age.

Assessment

Children and their parents attend an initial assessment before commencing treatment. The purpose of the assessment is to obtain a case history, diagnose stuttering, measure the severity of the child's stuttering, identify any other communication disorders, provide parents with information about stuttering and the treatment program, and begin developing rapport with the child and parents. In nearly all cases stuttering is easily diagnosed by consensus between the parents and clinician (Bloodstein, 1993). In rare cases where there is doubt about diagnosis, parents may be asked to provide additional recordings of their child's speech outside the clinic, or a second specialist clinician may be consulted so that consensus can be achieved.

The Basis of the Lidcombe Program

The Lidcombe Program incorporates operant methodology and is a parent-administered, early intervention program for stuttering. Response-contingent stimulation is applied in the form of praise for stutter-free speech and correction of stuttered speech. During 1-hour weekly clinic visits, each parent is taught to administer the treatment to his or her preschool child and to measure the severity of the child's stuttering. The components of the Lidcombe Program are parent training, speech measures, praise for stutter-free speech, correction of stuttered speech, problem solving, and maintenance. Each of these components is described below.

Speech Measures

The Lidcombe Program involves within- and beyond-clinic collection of measurements of the child's stuttering. There are several purposes for these measures: obtaining an initial assessment of stuttering severity, setting treatment goals, evaluating progress, facilitating communication between parent and clinician, and, finally, making it easier for each parent gradually to take on responsibility for using the Lidcombe Program with his or her child (Onslow, 1996).

Percent Syllables Stuttered (%SS)

This measure is collected during each clinic visit by the clinician, usually at the beginning of the session. The clinician or parent plays and talks with the child for approximately 10 minutes while the clinician counts stutter-free and stuttered syllables. These numbers are then converted to a percentage of syllables that are stuttered. At our clinics we use a small electronic device for this counting and calculation. We use percentage of syllables stuttered (%SS) as one way to assess clinical progress, by comparing the frequency of the child's stuttering in the clinic from week to week. We also use %SS to set treatment goals. For example, later in the treatment process, children will be enrolled in the maintenance phase of the program when they are able to achieve, among other things, less than 1%SS in the clinic and in beyond-clinic speaking situations over several consecutive weeks.

With older clients, speech rate in syllables per minute (SPM) is also measured during each clinic session. However, we have not found that SPM adds useful information when using the Lidcombe Program with preschool-age children, so it is not measured.

Severity Ratings

Severity ratings (SR) are used by parents to measure the severity of their child's stuttering in everyday situations outside the clinical setting. Parents rate the severity of their child's stuttering on a 10-point scale (1 = no stuttering, 10 = extremely severe stuttering). At the first clinic visit, the clinician explains the scale to the parents and asks them to graph the child's SRs on a chart each day for the following week. The parent can either give a global SR for the whole day or give an SR for a particular 10-minute period each day. If the second method is used, the parent is asked to identify seven of the child's everyday speaking situations. These may include, for example, meal times, in the car after preschool, or playing with friends. The parent is asked to rate a different situation each day. At each clinic session, the parent and clinician discuss SRs from the previous week. The clinician monitors the SRs for fluctuations in stuttering severity, evidence of generalization of treatment gains, and to better understand how treatment is progressing for each child and family.

The clinician assesses the agreement between the parent's and clinician's SRs during each clinic session. This is accomplished in the following manner. After the clinician collects %SS from the child's conversation in the clinic, the parent and clinician each assign an SR to it. The parent and clinician are considered to have acceptable agreement if their ratings are equal or within one scale value. If they do not meet this criterion, the discrepancy in ratings is discussed and resolved. Acceptable agreement between the parent and clinician ensures that they can communicate clearly about the child's speech using the SR scale (Onslow et al., 1990).

Stutters per Minute of Speaking Time (SMST)

Parents make 5- to 10-minute recordings of their child's speech in conversation from time to time. If the parent is using the SR scale on a 10-minute speaking situation each day, one of those situations can be recorded each week. The parent listens to the recording, counts the number of stutters in the sample, and measures with a stopwatch the length of the child's speaking time. The parent gives these measures to the clinician, who calculates SMST by dividing the speaking time by the number of stutters. During initial clinic visits, the clinician also collects an SMST measure from the parent's recordings for comparison. When the parent and clinician achieve acceptable agreement the clinician no longer checks the parent's measures. Agreement is judged to be acceptable when the parent's and clinician's SMST measures differ by no more than 5%.

At each clinic session the clinician charts the within- and beyond-clinic speech measures and discusses with the parent how well the measures represent the child's speech during the previous week. If the measures are not representative, then the situations in which beyond-clinic measures are collected may be changed. For example, the clinician may ask parents to collect SR and SMST measures only in speaking situations in which the child continues to stutter. The parent and clinician also discuss trends in the speech measures and their implications for progress. For example if a child's %SS and SR measures are decreasing, the clinician might begin preparing the parent for the maintenance phase of treatment.

Treatment Formats

Parents and clinicians administer treatment in two formats: sessions and on-line.

Sessions

"Sessions" refer to 10- to 15-minute games that the parent and child play together each day. The primary aim of these games is for the child to speak in effortless, consistently stutter-free speech. The parent introduces the child to the game and explains the goal, for example by saying, "While we are looking at this book, let's see if you can say lots of smooth words. When I hear smooth talking I'll say, 'Great talking.'" Stutters can be corrected during these sessions, but if the parent structures the session correctly, very few stutters will occur.

The activities used during treatment sessions are varied according to several factors, including (a) the severity and frequency of the child's stuttering, (b) the child's speech and language development, and (c) the child's interests. An example of a highly structured activity for a child with severe stuttering would be naming flash cards, while an unstructured activity for a child with mild stuttering would be playing with construction blocks. The aim of varying the structure of sessions is to ensure that the child produces predominantly stutter-free speech. It follows, therefore, that as the child's stuttering decreases, the parent decreases, among other things, the structure of therapy sessions at home.

Generally, children participate in one or two treatment sessions at home per day. Each session lasts for 10 to 15 minutes. For some children and parents, for example, very young children, children with short attention spans, children who stutter severely, or parents with more than one young child at home, it may be preferable to have two shorter sessions per day. We suggest to parents that they conduct therapy sessions in mornings or early afternoons, when preschool-age children are best able to cooperate with and benefit from them. We also suggest that parents avoid doing treatment sessions at bedtime, as the child will not experience any benefit from generalization.

As treatment progresses and the severity of the child's stuttering decreases, the number of sessions conducted each week is reduced. On-line feedback (see below) then becomes the predominant treatment format. At some point, usually around the time the child begins the maintenance program, treatment sessions cease and only on-line therapy is used.

On-line

On-line therapy refers to praise for stutter-free speech and correction of stuttered speech that occurs in everyday speaking situations. An example of on-line therapy would be when a parent detects a stutter in the child's speech while they are shopping and asks the child to correct the stutter. Another example would be when a parent comments to the child about smooth talking while playing in the park. The parent varies the timing frequency, and type of on-line therapy that the child receives throughout the day. These variations in on-line therapy are discussed and planned by the parent and clinician during weekly clinic visits.

Generally, on-line praise for stutter-free speech is introduced by the clinician when parents demonstrate that they can correctly identify stutter-free and stuttered speech during therapy sessions. This means that on-line praise is likely to be used by parents in conjunction with structured therapy sessions. On-line correction of stuttered speech is introduced when a child's stuttering is reducing in severity and both child and parent are comfortable with correction.

Treatment Targets

There are several treatment targets in the Lidcombe Program. Each of these targets is manipulated through response-contingent stimulation.

Stutter-Free Speech

Periods of stutter-free speech are praised and rewarded by the parent and clinician. Children receive praise such as, "Good talking," "Your speech sounds great," or "Your words are very smooth." The parent takes care to ensure that the praise is enthusiastic and sincere. Praise is sometimes combined with tangible reinforcers such as stickers or tokens. Tangible rewards are also used to increase children's motivation and to maintain their interest when doing structured therapy. For children who experience high levels of stuttering, one or two stutter-free words may be reinforced. For children who experience low levels of stuttering, two or three sentences of stutter-free speech may be reinforced. The expectations for stutter-free speech are reviewed on a daily basis and adjusted as necessary, depending on the child's capabilities on that day. In other words, the parent's expectations of stutter-free speech are adjusted to ensure that the child has many opportunities to receive positive feedback. The severity of preschool children's stuttering is highly variable, so treatment is tailored for each child on each day. This ensures that the child always achieves success during the therapy activity, regardless of stuttering severity. Care is always taken to ensure that each child receives far more praise than correction during both sessions and on-line therapy. Parents are advised to praise many more episodes of stutter-free speech than they make requests to correct stuttering. This balance minimizes the possibility that children are overwhelmed by feedback about their stuttering.

Stuttering

The goal of the Lidcombe Program is to eliminate stuttered speech. If the child stutters, the parent responds in one of the ways described below and then encourages the child to continue talking. At all times correction is presented in a natural and supportive manner, using a neutral tone of voice. It is important that there is no suggestion of anger or frustration from the parent. The following are examples of what a parent might do or say following a stutter:

- The parent ignores the stutter and continues with the conversation.
- The parent comments to the child that a "bumpy word" occurred and goes on with the conversation.
- The parent provides a correct model of the stuttered word and goes on with the conversation.
- The parent comments to the child that a "bumpy word" occurred and asks the child to repeat the word correctly.
- The parent asks the child to repeat the stuttered word correctly and when this occurs asks the child to repeat the stutter-free word once or twice more. Each successful reiteration is praised. This technique encourages overlearning of the correct production and increases the opportunities for the child's stutter-free speech to be praised.

Sometimes we work with children who are sensitive to having their stuttered speech corrected, particularly at the beginning of the treatment process. If this is the case, then treatment can proceed without correction of stuttered speech, but progress is likely to be slower. We find that correction of stutters can gradually be introduced after the child has had several weeks of only praise for stutter-free speech. With all children, parents and their clinicians consult each week about the frequency and type of correction used, and treatment is structured so that correction is kept to a minimum.

Self-Monitoring

Once children have had several weeks of treatment, they are praised and rewarded for correctly identifying their stutter-free speech. During sessions and on-line therapy a child might be asked, "Was that smooth?" and then reinforced for the correct answer. Similarly if a child identifies stutter-free speech without prompting, praise is also given. Often the first sign of the development of self-monitoring skills is self-correction of a stutter without prompting from the parent or the clinician.

Maintenance

The maintenance of stutter-free speech is also a treatment target. Maintaining stutter-free speech can be rewarded in a number of ways. The maintenance program schedule rewards the maintenance of stutter-free speech by decreasing the frequency of clinic visits. The parents of preschool children often find this more rewarding than do the children. The children enjoy coming to the clinic and playing and talking with the clinician.

Problem Solving

Throughout the treatment program, parents are encouraged to give the clinician feedback about the implementation of the program. A collaborative relationship develops in which the parent is the expert about the child and the clinician is the expert about the Lidcombe Program. The parent's input into clinic discussions is encouraged and respected, because it is necessary for the effective delivery of treatment. The parent and clinician work together to find the most effective way of conducting treatment for the child. Joint problem solving also increases the parent's skills in making decisions about the child's speech. This ability to problem-solve about the child's treatment assists successful long-term maintenance. Although many problems can occur during the course of treatment, the following are two examples to illustrate how they might be managed:

- A parent reports that the child is a little shy and becomes reluctant to talk when the tape recorder is turned on. The parent and clinician work out some situations where it will be possible to make covert recordings of the child's speech at home.
- A parent reports that the severity of the child's stuttering was consistently 2 throughout the previous week, except that it went up to 5 when they visited a friend's house. The parent is not sure whether to give on-line feedback to the child in front of friends. The parent

and clinician confer and agree that the parent will prompt the child about stutter-free speech in the car on the next visit to the friend's house and discreetly give the child some positive feedback during the visit.

Parent Training

As stated earlier, the Lidcombe Program is administered by parents. They deliver the treatment in their child's everyday speaking environment. Consequently, parents receive extensive training in the administration of the program. During the first weeks of training, the clinician demonstrates during therapy sessions how to praise stutter-free speech and correct stuttered speech. Parents then attempt the same activities and the clinician gives them feedback. The clinician may also ask a parent to tape record therapy sessions at home. The clinician and parent together listen to the recordings, and the clinician gives feedback to the parent about treatment skills.

Parents need to acquire various skills to use during therapy sessions. They learn to:

- Maintain the child's attention and compliance with the therapy activity
- Conduct a suitable activity that evokes stutter-free speech
- Evoke conversational responses and respond to what the child says
- Monitor for periods of stutter-free speech and stuttering
- Correctly identify stutter-free speech and stuttering
- Deliver praise and correction accurately, immediately and consistently, and in a positive manner
- Prompt and praise the child's self-evaluation of stutter-free speech
- Be ready to use a variety of techniques when helping the child to correct a stutter
- Make on-line judgments about when to correct and when to ignore stuttering
- Watch for any signs of distress in the child
- Judge an appropriate ratio of praise and correction, and change it as needed for the child.

When parents reach the stage of the program where on-line praise and correction occur, parents also:

- Maintain appropriate praise and correction
- Monitor the child's everyday speech for stutter-free and stuttered speech
- Prompt and praise stutter-free speech in many everyday situations
- Correct stuttered speech gently, without disturbing the child's overall communication
- Keep the child interested in continuing, intermittent praise for stutter-free speech.

Maintenance

For most children, maintenance begins when the average of their daily SR at home is 2.0 or lower and within-clinic speech measures are less than 1%SS for 3 consecutive weeks. The maintenance program is based on one described by Ingham (1980) and consists of a series of clinic visits. At each visit, the parent reports on the child's speech during the preceding week. Typically, visits are spaced in the following manner: 2 weeks, 2 weeks, 4 weeks, 4 weeks, 8 weeks, 8 weeks, 16 weeks, and perhaps a final visit at 32 weeks. The maintenance phase of the Lidcombe Program, therefore, is a series of assessments of the child's speech. The clinician specifies the speech criteria for the child to maintain, that is, SR averaging 2.0 or lower, SMST 1.0 or less, and less than 1%SS in a conversation in the clinic.

If the child's speech meets these criteria, the child moves to the next visit on the maintenance schedule. If a child does not achieve the speech criteria at a maintenance visit, several things may occur. First, the parent and clinician discuss possible reasons for the increase in stuttering. Second, strategies for reducing stuttering are agreed on and the parent and clinician negotiate a time frame for this to happen (e.g., 1 or 2 weeks). The child and parent visit the clinic again at the end of this period, and if the child's speech meets criteria, they again progress through the maintenance schedule.

During maintenance, the clinician advises the parent how to reduce the amount of on-line feedback given to the child. The therapy is reduced gradually, with careful monitoring to ensure that the child's stuttering does not increase again. An example would be parents giving on-line praise several times a day, gradually reducing this to once or twice a day, and then to every second day. Maintenance also helps parents and clinicians to detect signs of relapse quickly and to act on these accordingly. Finally, the maintenance clinic visits provide an opportunity for ongoing support to the child and parent by the clinician. Long-term maintenance of stutter-free speech takes effort and commitment by the parent, and support from the clinician can help achieve it.

EVALUATION

Outcome of the Lidcombe Program

The outcome of the Lidcombe Program for stuttering in preschool children is described in four publications (Lincoln & Onslow, 1997; Lincoln, Onslow, & Reed, 1997; Onslow et al, 1990, 1994). Its outcome with school-age stuttering children is described by Lincoln, Onslow, Lewis, and Wilson (1996).

Onslow et al. (1990) reported outcomes of the Lidcombe Program with four preschool children. Data were gathered in a variety of speaking situations for 2 months before treatment and 9 months after treatment. In parent surveys, all parents reported "no stuttering" immediately post-treatment and at 9 months post-treatment. The reported treatment effects were established in 5 to 8 clinical hours. Following this study, Onslow et al. (1994) conducted another trial of the Lidcombe Program with 12 subjects. Data were collected for 2 months before treatment and 12 months after treatment. The subjects achieved a median of 1.0%SS for the entire 12-month post-treatment period. Surveys were sent to the parents of the children after completion of maintenance. The five parents who responded to the survey reported an average stuttering severity rating of 1 or 2 on a 10-point severity rating scale. Parents also reported that they continued to give on-line feedback occasionally (i.e., daily or monthly). The reported treatment benefits were achieved in 10.5 clinical hours.

Lincoln and Onslow (1997) reported the longer term outcome of treatment from the two studies previously described. This study provided outcome data from the children at 2- to 7-years post-treatment. Additionally, data were collected 1- to 4-years post-treatment on a comparable clinical population who received the same treatment. The subjects in this study were 43 children who had been treated for stuttering between 2 and 5 years of age. Parents were requested to make three 10-minute recordings of their child's speech each year for 3 years. Questionnaires were sent to the parents at the same time as the tapes. Near zero stuttering levels were achieved post-treatment and were maintained long-term. These results suggest that preschool-age children treated for stuttering may not need to re-enter treatment for up to 7 years after their initial treatment.

Taken together, the results of these three studies suggest that the Lidcombe Program is effective in reducing stuttering to near zero levels in both the short and the long term. This result was achieved for all subjects who completed the program and were available for follow-up in the long term. Of particular interest is the relatively short time required for treatment when compared with treatment times for adults who stutter. Also of interest are the reports by parents that they continued to provide on-line feedback in the long term. Perhaps this suggests that for some children control of stuttering continued to be reliant on parents' feedback. Lincoln et al. (1997) compared the speech of children who received the Lidcombe Program with the speech of children of the same age and sex who had never stuttered. First, the %SS of the two groups of children was compared; both groups attracted similar measures of %SS. Then the number of "stuttering" versus "not stuttering" judgments made by experienced clinicians and unsophisticated listeners on the same speech samples was compared. Children who had never stuttered were identified as "stuttering" significantly more than the treated children.

Lincoln et al. (1997) concluded that the Lidcombe Program resulted in speech that was comparable with that of children of the same age who had never stuttered. These results are in contrast to the adult stuttering literature, which contains consistent findings that the speech of adults who have been treated for stuttering can reliably be distinguished from that of normal speakers (e.g., see Metz, Schiavetti, & Sacco, 1990). Although the findings of the Lincoln et al. (1997) study are encouraging, further investigation is required to determine why the normal speakers were identified as stuttering more frequently than the children who had received the Lidcombe Program. It is possible that some qualitative differences existed in the speech of the two groups, which the study did not assess.

Research in Progress and Future Directions

At this time, several studies are under way on the Lidcombe Program. One project is investigating the contribution of its various components. It is possible that not all components are necessary for effective treatment with all children. It is particularly important to establish to what degree correction of stuttered speech is necessary. As mentioned earlier in this chapter, this component has the potential to distress young children, so if treatment is effective without it, that would be a preferable form of treatment. Preliminary data suggest that this will be a useful area of further research.

Another series of studies is under way to develop an effective method of delivering the Lidcombe Program to stuttering children who live in rural areas and have limited access to speech pathology services. Clinical staff of our treatment centers have successfully attempted several variations of distance intervention models based on the Lidcombe Program. The project

Other projects under way are an investigation of the effects of the Lidcombe Program on the language development of preschool stuttering children and a randomized, controlled clinical trial of the Lidcombe Program in several overseas speech clinics. Finally, a series of case studies is planned to apply the Lidcombe Program systematically to stuttering in adults. Initial results with two adults have been promising.

SUMMARY

- The Lidcombe Program is a parent-administered, early intervention for stuttering in preschool children.
- The Lidcombe Program's initial development was influenced by research on the effect on stuttering of response-contingent stimulation.
- The components of the Lidcombe Program are parent training, speech measures, praise for stutter-free speech and correction of stuttered speech, problem solving, and maintenance.
- To date, four empirically based publications have demonstrated the short-and long-term outcomes of the Lidcombe Program.

REFERENCES

Bloodstein, O. (1993). *Stuttering: Search for a cause and a cure.* Boston, MA: Allyn and Bacon.

Ingham, R. J. (1980). Modification of maintenance and generalization during stuttering treatment. *Journal of Speech and Hearing Research, 23,* 732–745.

Ingham, R. J. (1984). *Stuttering and behavior therapy: Current status and experimental foundations.* San Diego, CA: College-Hill Press.

Lincoln, M., & Onslow, M. (1997). Long-term outcome of an early intervention programme for stuttering. *American Journal of Speech-Language Pathology, 6,* 51–58.

Lincoln, M. A., Onslow, M., Lewis, C., & Wilson, L. (1996). A clinical trial of an operant treatment for stuttering school-age children. *American Journal of Speech-Language Pathology, 5,* 73–85.

Lincoln, M., Onslow, M., & Reed, V. (1997). The social validity of treatment outcomes of an early intervention for stuttering. *American Journal of Speech-Language Pathology, 6,* 77–84.

Martin, R. R., Kuhl, P., & Haroldson, S. (1972). An experimental treatment with two preschool stuttering children. *Journal of Speech and Hearing Research, 15,* 743–752.

Metz, D. E., Schiavetti, N., & Sacco, P. R. (1990). Acoustic and psychophysical dimensions of the perceived speech naturalness of nonstutterers and posttreatment stutterers. *Journal of Speech and Hearing Disorders, 55,* 516–525.

Onslow, M. (1996). *Behavioral management of stuttering.* San Diego, CA: Singular Publishing Group.

Onslow, M., Andrews, C., & Costa, L. (1990). Parental severity scaling of early stuttered speech: Four case studies. *Australian Journal of Human Communication Disorders, 18,* 47–61.

Onslow, M., Andrews, C., & Lincoln, M. (1994). A control/experimental trial of an operant treatment for early stuttering. *Journal of Speech and Hearing Research, 37,* 1244–1259.

Onslow, M., Costa, L., & Rue, S. (1990). Direct early intervention with stuttering: Some preliminary data. *Journal of Speech and Hearing Disorders, 55,* 406–416.

Reed, C. G., & Godden, A. L. (1977). An experimental treatment using verbal punishment with two preschool stutterers. *Journal of Fluency Disorders, 2,* 225–233.

6

The Stuttering Intervention Program

REBEKAH H. PINDZOLA

INTRODUCTION

The *Stuttering Intervention Program: Age 3 to Grade 3* (Pindzola, 1987) is a complete fluency management system particularly well-suited for preschool- and early school-age children. The *Stuttering Intervention Program* (SIP) contains procedures for assessing incipient stuttering, guidelines for parent counseling and training, a direct fluency management program for the child, and support materials for implementation in a school setting. The treatment program is founded on the principles of event consequation, physiological maneuvers, and linguistic manipulation.

Elements of SIP reflect the author's influence by others in the field of fluency and fluency intervention. Authorities have long recognized the link between utterance length, linguistic complexity, and the likelihood of fluency disruption in children. The program proceeds in a length-complexity hierarchy, from single words to utterances with multiple points of vocal reinitiation. In modifying behavior, SIP employs the notion of event consequation. The author believes that feedback and constructive criticism are central to learning new behaviors and replacing less desirable ones. In this sense, the program is less one of stringent operant conditioning and more one of cognitive reshaping.

SIP also was profoundly influenced by authorities who recognized that physiological changes in respiration, phonation, and articulation precipitate new-found fluency (Perkins, 1971; Shine, 1980a, 1980b; Webster, 1980). "Targets" achievable by adults were modified in SIP to metalinguistic levels appropriate for children. Also, these targets or physiological maneuvers were reduced to those intuitively primal for children's fluency.

The author's clinical skills and insights into early fluency intervention evolved from the mid-1970s into an organized program that was revealed regionally and nationally in 1984 (Pindzola, 1984a, 1984b). *The Protocol for Differentiating the Incipient Stutterer* (Pindzola & White, 1986) forms the initial component of SIP. Modifications to the entire diagnostic and treatment program resulted in the monograph's commercial publication in 1987 (Pindzola, 1987). Clinical endorsements and discussions of both the protocol and the SIP have been forthcoming (Culatta & Goldberg, 1995; Gordon & Luper, 1992; Healey, 1991; Shapiro, 1998). The SIP also was reviewed by Bernstein-Ratner and Dow (1992).

THE PROGRAM

The SIP guides the clinician in the collection of information, analysis of behaviors, and formulation of treatment-related activities. The four component parts of SIP are summarized in Figure 6–1.

Part I: Evaluating the Child

Explicit identification procedures that can help distinguish between beginning stuttering and normally disfluent speech constitute the initial component of SIP. First published independently as *A Protocol for Differentiating the Incipient Stutterer* (Pindzola & White, 1986), the protocol, now an integral part of SIP, is an appraisal tool that synthesizes existing knowledge into a unique format that guides clinical observations, data collection, and interpretation. A numerical rating scale is used in which behaviors rated as "normal" or "probably normal" are assigned the value of 1, "questionable" 2, and "probably abnormal" a value of 3.

The protocol contains four sections. First, auditory behaviors of the speaker are scrutinized and quantified; second, visual evidences of speaking difficulties are listed; and third, subjective feelings and reported information are ascertained as historical and psychological indicators of chronic stuttering. The fourth section allows the speech pathologist to summarize the available evidence and arrive at a diagnostic decision.

Part 1: Evaluating the Child
    a. Recognizing the incipient stutterer
    b. Microanalyzing behaviors
    c. Obtaining baseline data on extent and severity

Part 2: Involving the Parents
    a. Gathering information
    b. Identifying fluency disruptors and enhancers
    c. Counseling
    d. Involving parents to model fluency, managing episodes of stuttering, and facilitating fluency generalization

Part 3: Enhancing Fluency (Treatment)
    a. Improving fluency with strategies (slow, soft, smooth)
    b. Practicing through hierarchies of difficulties
    c. Building in generalization

Part 4: Implementing in the Schools
    a. Writing the IEP for the child
    b. Informing/involving the teacher

Figure 6–1. Overview of SIP.

The protocol is completed from a sample of the child's natural speech. All auditory and visual behaviors are observed during connected discourse. Concurrently, one may find it is possible to discuss openly the child's feelings about speech, and what happens when his or her "voice gets stuck."

Auditory Behaviors

The protocol first examines eight categories of auditory behavior to differentiate incipient stuttering from nonstuttering. Representative literature supporting each of the eight categories is discussed fully in the SIP manual and is summarized here.

Type of Disfluency.   The predominant type of disfluency used by a speaker influences listener judgments of normalcy and so is assessed on the protocol. A preponderance of interjections, hesitations, location of repetitions within the speech unit, presence of prolonged speech sounds, or speech attempts with coexisting physical signs of struggle affects the degree of fluency abnormality (Ryan, 1974; Yairi & Lewis, 1984).

Size of Speech Unit Affected.   The size of the speech unit affected by the disfluency affects listener judgments of normalcy and is assessed on the protocol. The distributions of repetitions of whole phrases, repetitions of whole words, and repetitions of part-words are each important, as are locations of hesitations or pauses. A rule of thumb suggested by Perkins (1971) is that the smaller the speech unit affected the more abnormal the disfluency.

Frequency of Disfluencies.   The frequency with which disfluent behaviors occur has long been recognized as important in the diagnosis of stuttering and in appraising its severity. Metraux (1950) and Van Riper (1982) provided classic examples of normal and abnormal rates of syllable repetitions. The presence of prolongations may indicate a fluency disorder, and Van Riper's (1982) frequency criterion continues to be useful in differentiating stuttering from nonstuttering on the protocol.

The overall rate of disfluency also may be used on the protocol to differentiate the normal speaking child from the child with incipient stuttering. Research from Adams (1977) and from Yairi and Lewis (1984) shaped the development of the protocol.

Duration of Disfluencies.   The duration of disfluency may be expressed in two ways on the protocol, either as number of times for repetitions or as length of time for prolongations. Adams (1977) stated that part-word repetitions of incipient stutterers consist of one to five reiterations (e.g. "b-ball" or "b-b-b-b-b-ball"). This is contrasted with the number of reiterations of nonstuttering children, which typically does not exceed three.

Van Riper's (1982) more stringent guidelines suggested that more than two syllable repetitions per word are abnormal, while less than two per word may be considered normal. Yairi and Lewis' (1984) findings on part-word repetitions of 2- and 3-year-olds are in agreement with Van Riper's guidelines. The number of reiterations detected in the sample is important in the protocol.

The average duration of prolongations is measured as a length of time. Riley's (1972, 1980) procedure is recommended for the protocol and Van Riper's (1982) data provide the basis for interpretation on the protocol.

Audible Effort. Vocal tension, pitch rise, and other audible signs of effort while speaking are generally not found among normally fluent speakers and are indicative of abnormality on the protocol (Adams, 1977; Bloodstein, 1981; Van Riper, 1982).

Rhythm/Tempo/Speed of Disfluencies. Van Riper (1982) provided clinical reports that normal disfluencies and perhaps very early stutterings are characterized by repetitions that preserve the normal rhythm and rate of speech. Not until the tempo of the reiterations speeds up or their rhythm becomes irregular and choppy is there substantial reason for concern. Therefore, rhythm and tempo are noted.

Intrusion of Schwa Vowel During Repetitions. Another feature that may distinguish the repetitions of stuttering from those of non-stuttering speakers is the perceived presence of the schwa vowel. Although Van Riper (1982) provided anecdotal evidence that stuttering repetitions often have the neutral vowel "schwa" intruding on the intended vowel, acoustic evidence to support this intrusion hypothesis seems lacking (Allen, Peters, & Williams, 1975; Montgomery & Cooke, 1976). Because some authorities continue to support its perceptual reality as indicative of defects in coarticulatory transitions and of chronic stuttering (Adams, 1978; Cooper, 1973; Stromsta, 1965; Van Riper, 1982), the presence of schwa vowel intrusion is indicated on the protocol.

Audible Learned Behaviors. Word substitutions and circumlocutions may be used to avoid feared words, postponement devices may consist of maneuvers to delay attempts on a feared word, and starting tricks may be used to assist in initiating feared words. These and other audible mannerisms often discriminate between stuttering and nonstuttering and, if detected, are marked on the protocol.

Visual Evidence

Visible signs of effort suggest to the listener that the act of speaking is unduly difficult. The excess tensing of muscles might also represent the speaker's attempts to "break an invisible hold" and force out the word. Whatever the motivation, such visible evidence is considered by listeners in judging speech normalcy. Furthermore, the presence of visible effort indicates that the child is aware of speaking difficulties, is trying to do something about the moments of difficulty, and that the disfluency has progressed in severity. The protocol assesses three areas that often provide visual evidence of stuttering.

First, the clinician lists all facial contortions and articulatory posturing observed. Second, the presence of any rhythmical head movements, conspicuous head jerks, and the more subtle head turnings to divert eye contact are noted on the protocol. Third, the involvement of the hands, arms, legs, feet, and torso in unusual or rhythmical movements may be associated with a stuttering block and so are important diagnostic observations.

Historical and Psychological Indicators

The subjective evaluations made by a speaker while experiencing speech disfluencies and in reaction to them are diagnostically important. The child's perceptions of the problem are explored whenever possible during protocol assessment. Additional information collected from parental reports, although subjective, is important, as are parental opinions of how the child views the speech problem. Also, as explained more fully in the SIP manual, the clinician ascertains the awareness and concern of both the child and the parents, as possible indicators of chronicity and/or treatment style.

Another indicator assessed on the protocol is "Length of Time Fluency Problem has Existed." The literature suggests that children exhibiting disfluencies for a longer period of time are more likely to (a) be stuttering rather than merely experiencing a period of normal disfluency, (b) have a chronic problem that resists spontaneous recovery, and (c) have a severe fluency problem. Child disfluency cases receiving "early" evaluations and intervention strategies have better prognoses for normal fluency.

The protocol seeks to ascertain the "Consistent Versus Episodic Nature of Problem." According to Bloodstein (1960), one of the best indicators that stuttering is "still in its most rudimentary form is that it appears for periods of weeks or months between long interludes of normal speech" (p. 367). Parental reports of chronic, day-to-day disfluencies would, however, be a danger sign and are assessed.

The child's "Reaction to Stress" may be diagnostically and therapeutically important, and specific observations are made on the protocol regarding changes in frequency and types of disfluency during stressful situations. The observations of Bloodstein (1960, 1994), Van Riper (1963), and Ryan (1974) underpin this aspect of the *Stuttering Intervention Program*. Additional areas of protocol assessment cover "Phoneme/Word/Situation Fears and Avoidances," "Familial History," and "Other Covert Factors."

Summary of Clinical Evidence and Impressions

The protocol provides a systematic procedure for making specific observations regarding speech fluency. It categorizes auditory and visual behaviors on a grid which guides the clinician to a determination of whether the behavior is normal, questionable, or likely to be indicative of stuttering. While failure in any particular category is not an indication of a fluency problem, the presence of a number of questionable symptoms suggests a possible disorder or at least the need to monitor the child's fluency. The presence of several abnormal auditory and visual behaviors would lead a clinician to a diagnosis of stuttering.

The numerical rating scale (1–2–3) used in the Auditory and Visual sections of the protocol yields a total score for the client. The third section of the protocol, Historical and Psychological Indicators, does not contribute to this total. The lowest possible score (indicating "normal" or "probably normal") is 14, whereas the highest (and "probably abnormal") is 42. Standardization studies suggest that a total score of 14–21 is within normal limits, while a score greater than 21 may be indicative of incipient or confirmed stuttering.

Part II: Involving the Parents

The program is designed around parental involvement, although it may be adapted for significant others. Parents are intended to be part of the total intervention program, and the SIP outlines procedures for such ideal circumstances. The use of program resources and tasks to involve parents are illustratively described in this section. Details necessary to execute the SIP are available in the manual (Pindzola, 1987).

The initial meeting with the parents serves several purposes. Collection of the case history data provides basic information pertinent to the diagnosis, and this meeting also begins the dialogue between parent and clinician. It is a true counseling session, from which many questions and responses will serve as a springboard for future counseling topics. In addition to gathering information pertinent to the protocol (for the Historical and Psychological Indicators section), the clinician can explore the nature of the child's stuttering problem by following the topics suggested in SIP's "Questions to Elicit Discussions During Parent Interview." Also during this first parent counseling session, SIP directs the clinician to explain the danger signs of stuttering, taking care to point out and discuss the symptoms present and not present in the child. The goal is to help the parents identify characteristics in their child, rather than telling them what has been observed; it is a discovery process. "Stuttering: Some Danger Signs" is a useful handout provided in SIP. Similarly useful information for parents can be obtained from films and publications by the Stuttering Foundation of America (Walle, 1974, 1975, 1977).

The second meeting with the parents provides further opportunity to educate them about the nature of stuttering. Discussions revolve around whether their child is developing the more severe, progressive symptoms. SIP describes this counseling session as information sharing, and the program provides various resource handouts. Additionally, the clinician encourages the parents to elaborate on their child, their child's behavior, and their verbal and nonverbal reactions. Using the "Parental Assessment of Comments to Their Child" contained in SIP, information learned provides guidance on how to deal with instances of disfluencies in the home. The literature is replete with contradictory advice on what parents should do when their child stutters (e.g., Cooper, 1979; Johnson, 1959). It may be fine to instruct the child to "slow down," but the clinician should be sure of this first. Parents are involved in experimenting with the child's response to various suggested parental strategies.

Counseling sessions provide time to thoroughly explain the treatment program the child will receive and to encourage parents' participation in the treatment, both at home and in the clinical setting. Discussions also center around the home situation: the current daily routine, behavior/discipline problems, sibling relationships, and conditions known to affect the child's speech (e.g., stress, pressures, excitement, rivalry for attention, etc.). Behavioral and nonspeech situations are explored, using materials provided in SIP, such as "Parental Suggestions—General Home Management." Related home and behavioral management concerns can be found in Zwitman's (1978) book. Implementation of these suggestions in the home environment is monitored.

In subsequent counseling sessions, specific speech management techniques are discussed and parents are provided with a copy of "Parental Suggestions: Models of Fluency" from the SIP. Some of the suggestions for parents to model include the use of short sentences, developmentally appropriate vocabulary, an unhurried rate of talking, and SIP fluency enhancing strategies. It is important to note that, although all such strategies are discussed and demonstrated, only those appropriate for the child are employed in the home environment.

Once active parental participation in treatment sessions has begun, daily 15-minute practice sessions at home commence. A parent-child conversation, reading/looking at story books, or playing a game provides a daily opportunity to practice the "new way of talking." Such formal practice cements learning and provides generalization of target usage to the parents and home environment. The practice is considered formal in that the parent regularly delivers consequent events, just as in treatment sessions. Constructive feedback and correct target use are expected in these formal practice sessions.

Part III: Enhancing Fluency (Treatment)

Treatment Premises

The SIP is based on the notion of direct, early intervention for the incipient stutterer. The directness of the approach involves manipulation of fluency and ample practice with fluency enhancing strategies. Practice in the clinical situation is undertaken in a variety of activities to engender enthusiasm and a desire for fluent communication. Practice with the parent is undertaken both within the clinical environment and at home. Generalization begins early.

Fluency is established and fostered through clinical control of three fundamental elements: (a) event consequation via an operant conditioning paradigm, (b) fluency enhancement via altered physiological speaking processes, and (c) linguistic manipulation to decrease the likelihood of a fluency disruption. Figure 6–2 depicts these three foundations for fluency inherent in the SIP.

Conditioning via Event Consequation.   According to operant theory, when a behavior is followed by certain events and so occurs more frequently, those events are known as reinforcers. The positive event or reinforcement used in SIP can be a smile of approval, the remark of "good" for a job well done, or a trinket. Fluent utterances increase substantially when reinforced, and a clinician using the SIP gives positive feedback often.

Immediate punishment of a disfluency decreases the amount of future disfluencies. SIP employs punishment in the form of feedback, a consequence that informs the child not to "do it like that anymore." The feedback may be a suggestion, a gentle rebuke, or an admonition such as asking the child to stop talking for a moment, or to slow down, or to stretch it out more, or to try

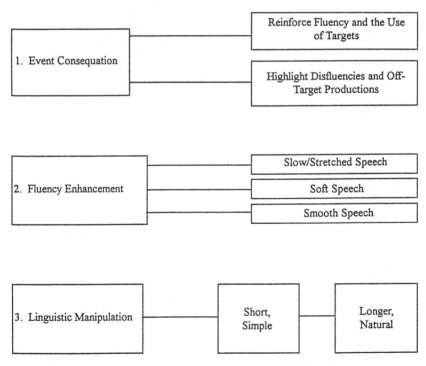

Figure 6–2. The SIP foundations for fluency. (From *Stutttering Intervention Program: Age 3 to Grade 3*, by R. H. Pindzola, 1987, p. 27. Austin, TX: Pro-Ed. Reprinted by permission.)

again, or simply a comment such as, "oops, that was a bumpy word." The information in the comment is constructive criticism. Throughout the SIP, stuttered responses are followed by the clinician saying "Oops," "Stop," or some equivalent feedback to the child as soon as a moment of stuttering is recognized—even before the child has completed the word. To be effective, the consequent feedback must be immediate.

After this brief stop, the child is allowed to begin again at that same word and employ any or all of the fluency strategies learned in treatment (such as stretching the first syllable of the utterance after having paused or breathed).

Fluency Enhancement Strategies.   Enhancing fluency constitutes a major portion of the SIP. Speech is the focus of treatment, and the child in the SIP is taught a "new way of talking" which involves three universal fluency enhancing strategies. These, for the sake of simplicity, are known as the "three S's": SLOW, SOFT, and SMOOTH speech.

The first fluency enhancer is slow, stretched speech. Stretched speech establishes immediate fluency and allows the vocal tract to stabilize and move slowly but deliberately through the first word (syllable) of the utterance. Materials for illustrative purposes include balloons, rubber bands, pieces of elastic, or Slinky toys. The client may manipulate the balloon in a stretching action while simultaneously practicing the verbal stimulus in a slow, stretched manner. The duration of the stretch is not critical in SIP; it is important to exaggerate the slowness and establish fluency. Practice stimuli begin with monosyllabic words, progressing to combined monosyllabic words, to polysyllables where only the first syllable need be stretched, to longer utterances, and eventually to spontaneous speech. It is important to note that, as the utterances lengthen, the slow stretching of speech is done only at points of vocal initiation, that is, at the beginning of sentences or following pauses. At these initiating and reinitiating points, only monosyllabic words and only the first syllable of polysyllabic words are to be stretched in this slow manner. This technique is different from the continuous slow pacing of many establishment programs (e.g., Shine, 1980b). The rationale is that because children who stutter tend to be disfluent mainly on the initial word of an utterance, only an initiation strategy is necessary and utilized in the SIP. This relatively unobtrusive target helps the child "get started" and allows resumption of a normal talking rate.

The second fluency enhancer is a soft speaking voice. Reduction of vocal loudness serves to reduce respiratory effort, decrease laryngeal tension, and preclude speech initiation with a hard glottal attack. This soft target is composed of two aspects in SIP. First, the client should reduce the overall loudness level and adopt a generally softer voice; and second, the client should exhibit a more pronounced loudness reduction on the syllable that is also to be stretched. In essence, this translates into an overall softer voice with extra softness on the first syllable of an utterance. Activities and stimuli progress in a manner similar to, and simultaneously with, the training of slow, stretched speech.

The third fluency enhancer encourages smooth-flowing speech where words within a breath group blend together. This is contrasted with choppy speech that lacks such smooth transitions. The child initially manipulates his or her index finger gently from crest to crest while talking. This manual movement can be likened to a pacing board, and further serves to establish fluency (Helm, 1979). The finger movement is initially done on a syllable-by-syllable basis, making this rhythmically paced speech highly fluent. Then, rather than pacing by syllables, which is highly artificial (e.g., al-li-ga-tor = 4 waves or beats), the child segments long words wherever it seems most appropriate (e.g., alli-gator = 2 waves or beats). This serves to maintain the normal rhythm of English and preserves syllable-to-syllable transitions in which breath and voice flow remain continuous within and between word boundaries.

Linguistic Manipulation.   The length and degree of difficulty of what a person says affect the probability that it will be fluent. Stuttering and nonstuttering children alike are more disfluent when saying long, difficult sentences. Consequently, by controlling a child's output, the clinician can affect the probability of fluency.

Early in treatment, when it is critical to ensure fluency, the clinician can "stack the deck" in the direction of fluency by allowing only short utterances. Utterances gradually lengthen when other fluency targets have been mastered in the program. In this regard the SIP is similar to other programs that control the length and complexity of utterances (cf. Costello, 1984; Ryan, 1974; Shine, 1980b; Stocker, 1976).

A Word About Treatment Activities

Step-by-step programming is provided in the SIP. However, clinicians are encouraged to adapt the program outline to the individual needs of the child. The SIP manual suggests a variety of treatment activities. The principle of generalization pervades the SIP activities and warrants special comment in this overview. By varying the speaking tasks, the activities of SIP begin the generalization process immediately. The newly acquired fluency must be transferred to all types of speaking activity, situations, and people frequently encountered in the child's life. The SIP builds in this generalization by practicing fluency targets in a variety of suggested speaking activities, by incorporating the parents and home practice early in the intervention process, and by altering verbal stimuli and linguistic contexts constantly during all sessions.

Throughout all treatment activities, the fluency targets should be practiced until they become habitual. Practice also includes maintaining fluency through target use in less than ideal situations. The real world contains social pressures, time pressures, and both positive and negative emotional upheavals. Treatment sessions provide practice in maintaining fluency and target usage while experiencing conditions of excitement. SIP incorporates such "pressure practice" in various activities to prepare the child for real world generalization of fluency.

Part IV: Implementation in the Schools

The speech-language pathologist working in the schools must not only service the child who stutters but also work within school board policies and procedures and with classroom teachers. Communication between the parents and the clinician is often infrequent. A close working relationship is therefore required with the classroom teacher to serve as an alternative source of information and to provide assistance in fluency practice. In return, the teacher expects help from the clinician with regard to classroom fluency management suggestions.

The SIP provides the speech-language pathologist with considerable assistance in these matters by including two Individualized Education Programs (IEPs). The child's "Present Level of Performance in Fluency" is based on the initial protocol data and any subsequent re-evaluation. The "Annual Goals and Short Term Objectives in Fluency" form is tailored to the SIP. The speech-language pathologist completes the necessary information for the IEP. The criterion for the annual goal must be determined for the child, and the specific therapeutic procedures and materials to be used should be stated for each objective. The short-term objectives of the SIP are listed in the order taught on the treatment outline. Achievement dates should be filled in to facilitate ongoing assessment of the child's progress. This streamlined "checklist and completion" format facilitates computerized case management.

The SIP also contains a "Teacher Information Packet" that is an ideal handout when conducting teacher in-service workshops. This information addresses topics most often of concern to a teacher with a child who stutters in the classroom.

EVALUATION

A series of statistical evaluations has been performed on the protocol. Estimates of reliability, validity, and normative reference points have been established and are described in the manual accompanying SIP. Some highlights are provided in this chapter.

A review of the literature of stuttering behaviors, danger signs, and guidelines for distinguishing normal from abnormal disfluencies resulted in a list of possible auditory and visual behaviors that should differentiate stutterers from nonstutterers. The resulting instrument, by definition of its formation, has content validity. The protocol's numerical rating scale, in which behaviors rated as "normal" or "probably normal" were assigned the value of 1, "questionable" 2, and "probably abnormal" 3, yielded numerical scores (both total and mean scores) and was used in further standardization studies.

The protocol was administered to 43 normal-speaking children aged 2 years, 7 months through 6 years, 4 months. The determination of normal speech was made on the basis of kindergarten teacher referral and screening for articulation, language, voice, fluency, and hearing by two speech-language pathologists as part of another study (Miller & Pindzola, 1985). Disfluent errors evident in the conversational speech samples of these children showed them to be "nonstuttering" by the absence of abnormal danger signs. Mean item scores, mean total scores, and total ranges of the normal children, by age group, using the protocol are presented in the SIP manual. Summary statistics indicate the item score averaged 1.24 and the total score averaged 17.3 for normal-speaking children. Normally speaking children in this standardization study did not exceed scores of 21.

Additionally, the protocol has construct validity for meaningful inferences, as measured by contrasting groups (Robb, Bernardoni, & Johnson, 1972): It adequately distinguishes between stutterers and nonstutterers. The protocol was administered to seven children referred for clinical evaluation of their disfluencies and for whom treatment was recommended. Seven normally fluent children, matched for age within 2 months, were randomly selected as control subjects. All subjects were between 2 years, 6 months and 10 years of age. Scores in the abnormal "danger" areas characterized the stuttering group's performance on the protocol, whereas the nonstutterers showed a preponderance of "probably normal" scores. In close agreement with the previous standardization study, nonstuttering children had a mean item score of 1.27; children who stuttered averaged 1.99. Of more importance, the mean total score on the protocol was 17.71 for the nonstuttering children as contrasted with 27.86 for the children who stuttered. Not only does inspection of these data indicate a difference between the group means, the 14 children displayed ranges of total protocol scores that do not overlap: Nonstutterers' total scores ranged from 15 to 20 and those of stutterers ranged from 22 to 40. These findings are in close agreement with the normative data from the previous standardization study.

Criterion-related validity was estimated using the concurrent validity method of test comparisons (Robb et al., 1972). This validity was tested by comparing the protocol scores with the *Stuttering Severity Instrument* (SSI) (Riley, 1972, 1980) scores for 11 stutterers. Pearson product-moment correlation was .92 for the total scores, suggesting a high relationship between the protocol's test content and its criterion. This .92 correlation proved significant at the .01 level (df = 2, critical value = .735), allowing conclusions to be made about the population of stutterers in general.

Pearson product-moment correlations between the protocol's 14 parts and the total score, and the correlations between the 14 protocol items and the SSI total scores also were obtained. These data are presented in the SIP manual. Items most highly correlated with the overall score of the protocol and with the SSI total score were type of disfluency, rhythm/tempo/speed of disfluencies, and the presence of audible learned behaviors. These items are therefore the most discriminating of the protocol.

To assess interjudge reliability among clinicians, a 15-minute videotaped sample of a stuttering child was examined by three experienced speech-language pathologists. Reliability correlations of .94 or greater were obtained for the total score, suggesting that the protocol is a reliable tool for clinicians to use in appraising stuttering.

Effectiveness measures for the parental component of the SIP have been determined. To document parental attitude change as a result of SIP counseling, the *Parental Diagnostic Questionnaire,* or PDQ (Tanner, 1978), was administered to the parents of three clients prior to and after the child's treatment program. According to Tanner, the mean values of sections 2 and 3 of the PDQ should decrease with improvements in parental attitude toward stuttering. Section 2 addresses attitudes of parents and their emotional reactions when the child tries to speak, and Section 3 queries the parents what they do or say when the child tries to speak.

Prior to receiving the parent counseling component of the Stuttering Intervention Program, the parents' mean score on Section 2 of the PDQ was 2.4, but following the counseling, the Section 2 mean score decreased to 1.3. This change represents improved parental attitudes.

Before counseling, the parents averaged 2.8 on Section 3 of the PDQ. After SIP parental intervention, the Section 3 score declined to a mean of 1.7, suggestive of improved parental reactions to the children's speech attempts.

The SIP and its treatment regimen have been in use for over 20 years. The authors and various professionals in a variety of work settings find its application simple and effective. Tightly controlled investigations of the therapeutic effectiveness of SIP are available for three preschool children; details appear in the manual. To summarize, pre- and post-treatment scores from the protocol showed an average overall improvement of 12 points. (Total protocol scores declined 13 points, 12 points, and 10 points, respectively, per child.) The mean total score prior to treatment for the children was 30.7; this declined to an average post-treatment score of 18.7.

More enlightening are the comparisons of certain pre/post measures within the protocol, notably frequency of stuttering and the occurrence of accessory behaviors. The amount of stuttering declined in all three children, as measured in two situations. The frequency of disfluencies in general was assessed prior to and at the termination of the SIP by the clinician in the therapeutic setting and by one parent in the home environment. Prior to intervention, child 1 exhibited 12% disfluency in the clinic and 15% in the home environment. A post-treatment assessment showed the same child to be 3% disfluent in the clinic and 0% at home. For child 2, disfluency decreased from 16% in the clinic and 23% at home to 7% in the therapeutic setting and 5% in the home. Disfluency rates in child 3 were likewise reduced from

11% in the clinic and 6% at home to 4% and 2%, respectively. In summary, the frequency of disfluency prior to and at the termination of SIP showed marked improvement for all children. On average, the percentage of disfluency declined 8.3% in the therapeutic setting, as measured by the clinician, and declined 12.3% in the home environment, as measured by a parent.

Diminution in the occurrence of accessory behaviors also is a good measure of improvement in terms of the disorder's conspicuousness to society. Scores from the following four protocol categories were combined to yield a general measure of accessory behaviors: audible effort, grimacing/articulatory posturing, head movements, and body involvement. Improvements made by the three clients through the SIP averaged 4.7 points; the average total protocol score for these four categories decreased from 8.7 to 4.0 as a result of treatment.

Parental perceptions provide valuable feedback on the fluency improvement of the child. The decline in stuttering and associated behaviors can be monitored, through the parent's eyes, by the PDQ (Tanner, 1978). A decline in the mean score from section 1 of the PDQ, administered before and after therapy, is suggestive of effective treatment. Prior to intervention, parents of these three clients averaged PDQ section 1 scores of 2.3, and following intervention SIP section 1 scores declined to a mean of 1.4, evidence of improved speech behaviors as observed by the parents.

SUMMARY

- The SIP is a complete fluency management system well suited for preschool and early school-age children.
- The Protocol for Differentiating the Incipient Stutterer investigates auditory and visual behaviors, and the historical and psychological indicators of chronicity.
- The Parent Counseling and Parent Training component of the SIP involves interviewing a parent and seeking and sharing information.
- The Direct Fluency Management component involves event consequation, fluency enhancement, and linguistic manipulation.
- The SIP is also implemented in schools with the involvement of teachers.

REFERENCES

Adams, M. R. (1977). A clinical strategy for differentiating the normally nonfluent child and the incipient stutterer. *Journal of Fluency Disorders, 2*, 141–148.

Adams, M. R. (1978). Further analysis of stuttering as a phonetic transition defect. *Journal of Fluency Disorders, 3*, 265–272.

Allen, C. D., Peters, R. W., & Williams, C. L. (1975, November). *Spectrographic study of fluent and stuttered speech.* Paper presented at the Annual Convention of the American Speech and Hearing Association, Washington, DC.

Bernstein-Ratner, N., & Dow, K. A. (1992). Therapy review. Pindzola, Rebekah (1987). The Stuttering Intervention Program (SIP). Tulsa: Modern Education Corporation. *Journal of Fluency Disorders, 17*, 283–290.

Bloodstein, O. (1960). The development of stuttering: II. Developmental phase. *Journal of Speech and Hearing Disorders, 25*, 366–376.

Bloodstein, O. (1994). *A handbook on stuttering* (5th ed.). San Diego, CA: Singular Publishing Group.

Cooper, E. B. (1973). The development of a stuttering chronicity prediction checklist for school age stutterers: A research inventory for clinicians. *Journal of Speech and Hearing Disorders, 38*, 215–223.

Cooper, E. B. (1979). Intervention procedures for the young stutterer. In H. Gregory (Ed.), *Controversies about stuttering therapy* (pp. 63–96). Baltimore: University Park Press.

Costello, J. M. (1984). Current behavioral treatments for children. In D. Prins & R. Ingham (Eds.), *Treatment of stuttering in early childhood: 1. Methods and issues* (pp. 69–112). San Diego, CA: College-Hill Press.

Culatta, R., & Goldberg, S. A. (1995). *Stuttering therapy: An integrated approach to theory and practice.* Boston: Allyn and Bacon.

Gordon, P., & Luper, H. (1992). The early identification of beginning stuttering: I. Protocols. *American Journal of Speech-Language Pathology, 1*(3), 43–53.

Healey, E. C. (1991). *Readings on research in stuttering.* White Plains, NY: Longman Publishing.

Helm, N. (1979). *Pacing boards.* Austin, TX: Exceptional Resources, Inc.

Johnson, W. (1959). *The onset of stuttering.* Minneapolis: University of Minnesota Press.

Metraux, R. W. (1950). Speech profiles of the pre-school child 18 to 54 months. *Journal of Speech and Hearing Disorders, 15*, 37–53.

Miller, M. K., & Pindzola, R. H. (1985, November). *The development of speaking rates in preschool children.* Paper presented at the Annual Convention of the American Speech-Language-Hearing Association, Washington, DC.

Montgomery, A. A., & Cooke, P. A. (1976). Perceptual and acoustic analysis of repetitions in stuttered speech. *Journal of Communication Disorders, 9*, 317–330.

Perkins, W. H. (1971). *Speech pathology: An applied behavioral science*. St. Louis, MO: C. V. Mosby.

Pindzola, R. H. (1984a, April). *The management of stuttering in the young child*. Paper presented at the Annual Convention of the Speech and Hearing Association of Alabama, Gulf Shores, AL.

Pindzola, R. H. (1984b, November). *Stuttering intervention: Age 3 to grade 3*. Paper presented at the Annual Convention of the American Speech-Language Hearing Association, San Francisco, CA.

Pindzola, R. H. (1987). *Stuttering intervention program: Age 3 to grade 3*. Austin, TX: Pro-Ed.

Pindzola, R. H., & White, D. T. (1986). A protocol for differentiating the incipient stutterer. *Language, Speech and Hearing Services in Schools, 17*, 2–15.

Riley, G. D. (1972). A stuttering severity instrument for children and adults. *Journal of Speech and Hearing Disorders, 37*, 314–320.

Riley, G. D. (1980). *Stuttering severity instrument for children and adults*. Tigard, OR: C. C. Publications.

Robb, C. P., Bernardoni, L. C., & Johnson, R. W. (1972). *Assessment of individual mental ability*. New York: Intext Educational Publications.

Ryan, B. P. (1974). *Programmed therapy for stuttering in children and adults*. Springfield, IL: Charles C. Thomas.

Shapiro, D. (1998). *Stuttering intervention: A collaborative journey to fluency freedom*. Austin, TX: Pro-Ed.

Shine, R. E. (1980a). Direct management of the beginning stutterer. *Seminars in Speech, Language and Hearing, 1*, 339–350.

Shine, R. E. (1980b). *Systematic fluency training for children*. Tigard, OR: C. C. Publications.

Stocker, B. (1976). *The Stocker probe technique*. Tulsa, OK: Modern Education Corp.

Stromsta, C. (1965). A spectrographic study of disfluencies labeled as stuttering by parents. *De Therapia Vocis et Loquelae, 1*, 317–320.

Tanner, D. (1978). *Parental diagnostic questionnaire*. Tulsa, OK: Modern Education Corp.

Van Riper, C. (1963). *Speech correction: Principles and methods* (4th ed.). Englewood Cliffs, NJ: Prentice-Hall.

Van Riper, C. (1982). *The nature of stuttering* (2nd ed.). Englewood Cliffs, NJ: Prentice-Hall.

Walle, E. (1974). *The prevention of stuttering: I. Identifying danger signs* [Film]. Memphis, TN: Speech Foundation of America.

Walle, E. (1975). *The prevention of stuttering: II. Parent counseling and elimination of the problem* [Film]. Memphis, TN: Speech Foundation of America.

Walle, E. (1977). *The prevention of stuttering: III. SSStuttering and your child, is it me? Is it you?* [Film]. Memphis, TN: Speech Foundation of America.

Webster, R. (1980). *Precision fluency shaping program*. Blacksburg, VA: University Publications.

Yairi, E., & Lewis, B. (1984). Disfluencies at the onset of stuttering. *Journal of Speech and Hearing Research, 27,* 154–159.

Zwitman, D. H. (1978). *The disfluent child: A management program.* Baltimore: University Park Press.

7

Speech Motor Training

JEANNA RILEY
GLYNDON RILEY

INTRODUCTION

History and Theory

A speech motor training program to treat stuttering was developed over 20 years based on empirical, theoretical, and research evidence. The possibility of a reduced speech motor system underlying stuttering was hypothesized. If a reduced speech motor system existed in a child who stuttered, the questions emerged, how to test it, how to train it? If speech motor function improved through training, would it have a positive impact on decreasing stuttering and/or providing a more effective speech motor system to support fluency? That is, when fluency was achieved, would a better speech motor system reduce the tenuousness of maintaining fluency? Also, would such a system eliminate the need for maintenance after treatment? It was from these questions that the speech motor program was developed. The available evidence, although inconsistent, provides a reasonable foundation for the hypothesis that in people who stutter some subsystems of speech motor production are reduced in efficiency and stability or, if functioning normally, do not interact appropriately. This hypothesized compromise of speech motor functioning may be a risk factor in developing stuttering because it has been noted in children as well as in adults. Also, children who stutter have longer manual reaction times than matched controls, suggesting that their motor differences are not limited to the speech system.

The theoretical framework underlying Speech Motor Training (SMT) was first elucidated by Stetson (1951). His research in motor phonetics led to a set of principles, including: (a) the syllable is the basic unit of speech production and (b) abutting speech sounds overlap (i.e., are coarticulated). Coarticulation has been described in more detail by Kent and Minifie (1977) and Sharf and Ohde (1981), among others. Models have been proposed that emphasize the constraints imposed by the speech production system so that output is not organized on a phoneme-by-phoneme basis (Liberman, Cooper, Shankweiler, & Studdert-Kennedy, 1967). Other models emphasize the importance of the intended target (MacNeilage, 1970) or temporal ordering (Lashley, 1951). It is assumed that speech motor training targets speech production planning, including functions that involve feed-forward controls.

Evidence in support of the role of open loop speech motor planning comes from several sources. Recently, acoustic studies using the F_2 formant transition have added specific details to the description of coarticulation (Liss & Weismer, 1992; Sussman, Hoemeke, & McCaffrey, 1992; Weismer, Kent, Hodge, & Martin, 1988). Lenneberg (1967), among others, described the enormous complexity of producing spontaneous speech using over 100 muscles and requiring thousands of neural events to produce up to seven syllables per second. He provided support from human and nonhuman studies of muscle control for the hypothesis that an open loop, feed-forward system assumed major responsibility for programming speech motor patterns. Goldberg (1985) described a medial loop as "projectional" and "feedforward," in contrast to a lateral loop that involves more on-line, feedback modifications during speech.

A variety of laboratory procedures, such as jaw tracking, kinematic measures of the relation of the upper lip and lip and jaw, can be performed with adequate reliability to provide an indication of the integrity of the speech motor system. Investigators often employ spectrographic measurement of acoustic durations of selected brief speech events. Vocal reaction time measurements are also used to provide evidence of the overall efficiency of the laryngeal systems. DeNil and Brutten (1991) reviewed studies of vocal reaction time (VRT) and acoustic duration (e.g., voice onset time [VOT]) and concluded that "there seems little doubt that stutterers have slower VRTs compared to normally fluent speakers" [p. 143]). The vocal reaction time studies with children who stutter seem to indicate differences between them and their matched controls. Seven studies of speech reaction time (SRT) included speech or vocal reaction times (vocal initiation time [VIT] or vocal termination time [VTT]); they reported significant differences between children who stutter, as a group, and the control groups (Bishop, Williams, & Cooper, 1991a, 1991b; Cross & Luper, 1979; Cullinan & Springer, 1980; Maske-Cash & Curlee, 1995; McKnight & Cullinan, 1987; Till, Reich, Dickey, & Seiber, 1983). Only one study (Murphy & Baumgartner, 1981) reported unequivocally that VRT was not significantly related to group (stuttering vs. controls) or to severity of stuttering. Cullinan and colleagues divided the children who stuttered into a "stutter plus" group, who were reported by their speech-language pathologists to have other speech or language problems in addition to stuttering, and a "stutter only" group, who had no additional problems. In their first study (Cullinan & Springer, 1980), the stutter-plus group accounted for the finding that stutterers were slower than their controls on both voice initiation time (VIT) and voice termination time (VTT). In the second study (McKnight & Cullinan, 1987), both stuttering groups had longer VTTs but only the stutter-plus group had longer VITs than the controls. Maske-Cash and Curlee (1995) replicated the Cullinan studies and concluded that the three groups, stutter only, stutter-plus, and controls, seemed to process and execute speech motor events differently. Three studies in which vocal reaction time and manual reaction time were combined reported that the children who stuttered had significantly longer manual reaction times than their controls (Bishop et al., 1991a, 1991b; Till et al., 1983; Williams & Bishop, 1992). In another study (Cross & Luper, 1983), finger reaction time (FRT) and VRT were highly correlated ($r = .92$). Thus, some significant slowing of reaction times was found in eight of the nine experiments reviewed.

Acoustic duration studies have produced ambiguous results. Healey and Adams (1981) found no consistent differences in temporal measures between children who stutter and controls. Wall, Starkweather, and Harris (1981) found no difference between stuttering frequency and duration of voiced to voiceless transitions. Zebrowski, Conture, and Cudahy (1985) found no differences favoring the control group in stop gap, voice onset time, (VOT), or other acoustic measures. They did report differences in the ratios between stop gap and aspiration, in that the controls exhibited an inverse relation between these two measures and the children who stuttered did not show any clear pattern. DeNil and Brutten (1991) reported that the VOTs of children who stuttered were not significantly longer but exhibited more variability than those of controls. Three studies have reported significantly longer VOTs for children who stutter (Adams, 1987; Agnello, Wingate, & Wendell, 1974; Howell, Sackin, & Rustin, 1995). The study by Adams was specifically designed to obtain a naturalistic sample of the children's speech tokens for analysis. Using five carefully matched stuttering subjects and five controls, Adams elicited phrase length speech samples with the tokens embedded in the phrase which was perceptually free of stuttering. The children who stuttered had longer VOT measures than the controls. Adams suggested that the use of tokens embedded in a repeated carrier phrase may improve timing characteristics of speech in children who stutter. Howell et al. compared six 7- to 10-year-old children who stuttered severely to six controls. They found that children who stutter (CWS) had significantly longer VOTs than the controls following /k/ and /t/ but not following /p/. Differences in subject selection criteria between studies (severe vs. mild-moderate) and the types of tokens selected may account for contradictory findings in the studies of acoustic durations in CWS.

Howell et al. (1995) also found significant differences between CWS and fluent controls in a jaw tracking task. They reported that the CWS "show roughly twice the tracking error as the fluent speakers for the lower lip and jaw" (p. 250). The CWS group made minimal displacement of the lower lip with the aid of visual feedback that was three times greater than the controls; without feedback, this difference increased to 4.6 times greater than the controls.

Kloth, Janssen, Kraaimaat, and Brutten (1995) obtained speaking samples from 93 preschool children prior to the onset of stuttering. These "high-risk" children came from families in which one or both parents stuttered. One year later, 26 of the 93 children had begun to stutter. The children who developed stuttering had receptive and expressive language skills equivalent to the children who did not develop stuttering; however, the CWS had significantly faster articulation rates. The authors speculated that the fast articulation rate among the CWS places unacceptable pressure on their marginal or even normal speech production system.

If reduced speech motor production ability is hypothesized as a risk factor for developing stuttering, then improvement of speech motor control is a legitimate target of stuttering treatment. SMT was designed to improve motor planning of syllable production in children who stutter. SMT has five features that recommend it as a treatment choice for young children who stutter:

- Improved motor timing and sequencing to support fluent speech should prevent or slow the development of stuttering and reduce overall treatment duration
- The use of nonlinguistic syllables requires no self-monitoring of stuttering events by the child
- Breath control does not involve cognitive training
- SMT provides a foundation to aid in maintaining fluency after it is achieved
- Post-therapy speech naturalness is not a problem because artificial speech is not induced in conversational speech.

Development of the Program

Oral Motor Training was devised to provide a systematic program to improve syllable production characteristics (voicing, coarticulation, and sequencing). Its use with children who stutter was based on the clinical observation that stuttering was reduced by a phonetic generalization program (McDonald, 1964) in children who had both stuttering and articulation problems. McDonald applied the basic principles of motor phonetics (Stetson, 1951) to articulation therapy. The syllable is considered to be the basic unit of speech production, just as the phoneme is the basic unit of perception of speech. Abutting phones overlap (are coarticulated) so that the phonetic environment influences the production of each sound. Given the complexity of neuromotor coordination and the speed of speech production (three or more syllables per second), the concept of a "feed-forward" (or open-loop) system was added to the feedback (or closed loop) system to help account for a child's ability to produce fluent, intelligible speech (see Borden, Harris, & Raphael, 1994, pp. 157–170 for review).

The third revision was published as *Oral Motor Assessment and Treatment: Improving Syllable Production* (Riley & Riley, 1985). The version in this chapter was revised during a 4-year, carefully controlled, funded investigation.

THE PROGRAM

The purpose of SMT is to improve speech motor production, thus reducing stuttering frequency and severity. Improvement in speech motor control can be inferred from changes in VRT and durations of brief acoustic speech segments following treatment. These changes in speech motor production are reported from controlled experimental studies but cannot be measured in most clinical applications. The behavioral goal of SMT is that the child will produce complex sets of syllables with correct voicing/unvoicing, smooth airflow, correct sequencing, and at an age-appropriate rate.

Clinicians who are planning to use the SMT program need to (a) develop the required clinical skills, (b) learn the general principles of training (including handling special problems) so that they are readily applied during the training sessions, and (c) follow specific training procedures that implement the principles on which this therapy is based.

The equipment required includes a good tape recorder, a high-quality external microphone, and a stop watch.

Clinical Skills Required to Recognize Abnormal Syllable Production

1. *The clinician must learn to recognize the characteristics of normal and abnormal syllable production.* Normal speech is smooth and connected. If a child says "He - hit - the - ball" in a disconnected way, the speech sounds abnormal. It seems like staccato talking. Smooth flow sounds natural when the child is saying strings of syllables. In SMT, the clinician models a group of syllables in a smooth, coarticulated manner and rewards the child for following the example. The groups of syllables that the clinician models are referred to as "sets." For example, /ba/ would be a one-syllable set, /mouta bu/ would be a three-syllable set. In a coarticulated production of the three sets /vami vami vami/ there should be no airflow breaks even between the sets. A better written transcript would be /vamivamivami/. Abnormal breaks can occur anywhere, for example, /va-mivamiva-mi/ or /vami-vami-vami/. A clinician preparing to use SMT should practice saying the sample syllable training sets described in the Outline of SMT (Table 7–2). Each set should be produced at least five times in a smooth, coarticulated manner, and recorded on audiotape. By repeated listening to the recording, the clinician can discover any airflow disruptions. The clinician can also practice pro-

ducing strings of sets with intentional airflow breaks to observe their abnormal sound and feel. After listening to these errors, it becomes easier to hear the child's airflow breaks.

2. *The clinician should be trained to recognize voicing errors.* They are somewhat less discernible during syllable repetitions. For example the v/f might be missed in /fami fami vami vami/. The repeated syllable set should be tape recorded and the v/f substitutions identified.

3. The clinician needs to be trained to recognize sequencing errors. An example would be when the target set is /vami/ and the child says /miva/ (transposed), /vava/ (repeated first syllable), or /va/ (omitted second syllable).

4. *Changes in rate of syllable production are an integral part of SMT.* The clinician needs to use a stop watch and make a tape illustrating different training rates. This practice tape should include syllable productions at 1 syllable per second (sps), 2 sps, and 3 sps (normal rate for young children). For example, if the production of /vami vami vami/ at 1 sps is taped, the total time will be 6 seconds. If the rate is increased to 2 sps, the total time will be 3 seconds. When the sets are spoken at a normal rate for a child (3 sps), the total time will be 2 seconds. These different rates should be practiced until they are automatic. The rate should be reviewed every 2 weeks because there is a tendency to revert to a faster rate.

5. *The syllable production model should be given without explanation.* Often, there is a natural instinct to "teach" the child rather than model a behavior. For reasons that are explained in the next section of the program, the child is to practice at the automatic level and not think about it. Table 7–1 provides examples of appropriate and inappropriate responses on the part of the clinician.

General Principles of Training

1. Motor training should be done at three rates: very slow (1 sps), slow (2 sps), and normal (3 sps). One sps

Table 7–1. Examples of the syllable production method.

Clinician	Child	Clinician
(Stimulus: clinician models correct production)	(Response: Child tries to repeat as per clinician's model)	(Reinforcement: based on child's production, clinican says "right" and gives token or says wrong" and withholds token.)
Listen, say /vami/ [at 1 sps].	/vami/. [at normal rate of 3 sps]	Wrong [because of fast rate] let's try it again. [withholds token]
Say /vami/ [at 1 sps].	/vami/ [at 1 sps]S.	Right. [+ token]
Listen, say /vamivamivami/.	I can't say that.	[Clinician's inappropriate response:] You need to say it to help you learn to talk. [explanation isn't needed]
		[Clinician's appropriate response]: OK, try this.
Say /vamivami/.	/vamivami/.	Good. [+ token]
Now, say /vamivamivami].	/vamivamivami/.	Good. [+ token]

and then 2 sps are the training rates; a rate of 3 sps is used in the last phase of training a given set.

2. After a given set at the same level of difficulty has been accurately trained, probing for generalization is done at an age-appropriate rate of approximately 3 sps. A set that is new to the child and is at the same level of difficulty is selected. For example, if /vami/ has been trained, the set /bounu/ could be used as a probe for generalization because it has two syllables in a CVCV configuration and the consonants are all voiced.

3. Training is done by modeling the desired behaviors. Instruction is used only when absolutely necessary. Speech motor performance is faster than children can think, so asking children to think about what they are doing interferes with normal motor planning. For example, breathing takes very little time, but thinking

"take a breath" and then performing the task takes much more time; so the clinician should model a good breath without further instruction.

4. Varying syllable stress is modeled during SMT to improve the flow of nonlinguistic syllables. The stress patterns make the exercise more like real speech. Two-syllable sets can be stressed on the first or second syllable (e.g., /ba' tou/ or /ba tou'/; three syllable sets can be stressed on the first, second, or third syllable.

5. Vowels, /i/, /æ/ /eɪ,/ /ou/, /u/, /a/, /aɪ/ were selected for inclusion in the training sets because they seemed natural and easy to produce. Sometimes children whose native language is not English find that some vowels are more comfortable than others. These children should be permitted to change to any vowel that makes the set easier to produce.

Specific Training Procedures

1. The levels of difficulty of SMT are indicated in the Outline of Speech Motor Training (see Table 7–2). Note that there are 14 levels of difficulty, from Level 1 (e.g., /mou/) to Level 14 (e.g., /mi tan gu aet/).

2. For each set indicated, the number of times the syllable set is modeled by the clinician and then produced by the child in one breath group is varied systematically: first one set is produced in a breath group (e.g., /bavi/), then 2 sets in a breath group (e.g., /bavibavi/), then 3 sets, then 5 sets, then 8 sets, and then 10 sets (e.g., /bavibavibavibavibavibavibavibavibavibavi/). For long strings of sets with three and four syllables, the child may need to take an extra breath.

3. The rate is varied systematically. At first, one syllable per second is used. For example, a three-syllable set will require 3 seconds to model and 3 seconds for the child to perform. This rate is not comfortable, but it requires practice to model at this rate and to assist the child to maintain it. Rate is increased to 2 sps then 3 sps as the child progresses through training on the selected syllable set.

4. Accurate voicing (unvoiced or voiced) and smooth flow are maintained. A child can usually produce voiced consonants more easily than the unvoiced cognates. So /zi zi zi zi/ is easier to say than /si si si si/. Therefore, when voiceless consonants are used in a training set, it is important to monitor correct voicing. SMT requires the child to produce a flow of syllables coarticulated across phoneme and syllable boundaries. This type of coarticulation replicates normal speech. Very brief airflow breaks can be detected between syllables that are not coarticulated. Clinicians need to practice listening for these breaks so that syllable flow is reinforced only when it is correctly coarticulated. The syllable sets should be initiated in an easy manner.

5. Contingency management can be used (tokens, moves in a game, points toward a backup reinforcer such as a toy). The reinforcement schedule can be designed by the clinician as long as it is consistently applied and the child is willing to work for the reinforcer. Contingency contracting using play time is useful to maintain a good response production. A sample ratio is 3–7 minutes drill to 5 minutes play.

6. The pass criterion at each step for a training set is three consecutive successes. The level (description of level is provided under Specific Training Procedures) is passed when a child can perform the trained set and two untrained sets; 80% accuracy is required to pass (i.e., 8 of 10 sets must be correctly performed).

7. If a child fails to perform correctly on six consecutive tries, he or she should branch to an easier level. For example if a child fails /moutabi/, branch to /moudabi/ (reduces complexity by using all voiced consonants). If the child fails three sets at the first level, some easier motor training program or special techniques should be used to get past this difficulty.

8. The clinician and child establish a pattern of training during Level 1 that will influence all other levels. It is important to adhere to the strict definitions of smooth flow and coarticulation as well as accuracy and rate. The clinician should not move to the next level until the child's production is automatic and overlearned. The very young child requires more training at Level 1 than older children.

Special Problems

1. *Breath control is a problem for about half of the children who receive SMT.* If the child is having trouble following the clinician's breath intake model, it may be necessary to branch to specific training in breath control. The clinician should highlight the breathing by pointing to the mouth. First, just model a breath followed by a single easy syllable; then model a breath followed by two syllables, then three syllables. Next model breath, syllable, breath, syllable, so the child must insert the second breath after a brief delay. Continue to lengthen this exercise until the child can follow the model: five syllables, breath, five syllables. If the child exaggerates the breath intake, model short, easy breath intake and do not reinforce the longer intakes used by the child. Verbal instruction is seldom required. If the clinician says, "take a deep breath" or "take a quick, deep breath," the child must move breath control to the cognitive level. The child needs to be able to sustain syllable production for 15 seconds to perform some of the SMT exercises. Sometimes a child will sigh, cough, or clear the throat prior to speaking. These behaviors may exhale the air in the lungs and the child may try to talk on reduced air supply. If this happens, model a sigh, breath, syllable so the child learns to take a breath just prior to syllable production.

2. The child may stutter during SMT. Stuttering is rare during SMT because the use of slow speech after modeling usually produces fluent syllables. If stuttering occurs, the clinician should say the set along with the child. This choral speaking effect usually eliminates the stuttering.

Levels of Difficulty

As shown in Table 7–2, there are 14 levels of difficulty provided for SMT. These levels are based on three variables: (a) the number of syllables in the set, (b) the number of unvoiced consonants in the set, and (c) the shape of the syllable set (CV, VCV, VCCV, etc.). The 14 levels were selected to represent a wide range of

Table 7–2. Outline of Motor Speech Training.

Levels	Training	Probing
Level 1 Single syllable, CV, all voiced	mo ve ba	ma zi bæ
Level 2 (optional) 1 syllable × 2 CV, all voiced	ni ni mu mu bo bo	mæ mæ go go zu zu
Level 3 2 syllables, CVCV, all voiced	wi ve val bu ma go	go mo næ wa vu ge
Level 4 1 syllable, CV, unvoiced	fi se kai	to pæ si
Level 5 2 syllables, CVCV, 1 unvoiced	mæ fi tu ne zi pe	val pe wu fo tæ gu
Level 6 2 syllables, VCV, all voiced	a vu e dæ u gi	aɪ zo o bo o zi
Level 7 2 syllables, VCCV, 1 unvoiced	um ku æp nai ib su	ot vu af do æn sa
Level 8 2 syllables, VCCV, 2 unvoiced	if pe at fi ok si	of tu af to up saɪ
Level 9 (optional) 3 syllables, CVCVCV, 2 syllables same, all voiced	wi va ve va mu ve du ni ni	mu mi go go va væ za mo mo
Level 10 3 syllables, CVCVCV, all voiced	næ za mi bi ma du ze wa mi	zu du wa nu be ni ga wu me

Table 7–2. *(continued)*

Levels	Training	Probing
Level 11 3 syllables, CVCVCV, 1 unvoiced	mi ta bo pe nu va ga wi fu	za ko mi va ko mu be va so
Level 12 3 syllables, CVCVCV, 2 unvoiced	mi ta po se va fi væ se ki	pa gu pi mo ta fu ko du fi
Level 13 3 syllables, CVCVCV, all unvoiced	fo ka to su to fi pa so tu	fe su ka tu pi fe ka su po
Level 14 (optional) 4 syllables, varied syllable shapes: V, CV, VC, CVC	si u ve mad wou kin da ik pev me tou nu	uf aɪ za nab mi tan gu æt kæt san ta fus

speech motor challenge. For each level there are three Training Sets and three Probe sets. Syllable sets are written in phonetic transcription without markers except that, for clarity, /ou/ is written as /o/ and /eɪ/ as /e/. The vowel code adapted from IPA is: /i/ as in beet; /æ/ as in bat; /e/ as in mate; /o/ as in boat; /u/ as in boot; /a/ as in hot; /aɪ/ as in might.

EVALUATION

Reduction in Stuttering

Riley and Riley (1986, 1991) conducted a retrospective study of nine children aged 3.3 to 6.8 and reported that stuttering had been reduced 19–100%. A prospective pilot study of three children aged 4.9 to 9.7 showed stuttering reduced by 37–70%. These data led to the decision to observe SMT effects in a more systematic, controlled experiment with a pre- and post-treatment design (Ingham & Riley, 1998). Percent syllables stuttered data were collected within and beyond the clinic during a 12-week baseline condition and during an 8-week withdrawal condition. The Stuttering Prediction Instrument (Riley, 1981) was also administered during baseline and withdrawal. This instrument employs parent interview and clinical observation to assess (a) the child's *reactions* to disfluencies, such as frustration, physical struggle, word avoidance, and teasing; (b) the characteristics of the types of disfluency observed, such as amount of tension and number of part-word repetitions, duration of prolongations and tense pauses; and (c) the frequency of stuttering in words stuttered per 100. Table 7–3 shows the characteristics of six children who participated in the Ingham and Riley study, at the beginning of treatment. Table 7–4 shows the observed changes for each dependent variable for each individual and for the group.

Note that four of the six children had significant reduction in stuttering frequency in both clinic and beyond clinic settings; one improved significantly only within the clinic and one only beyond the clinic setting. Group data show that all dependent variables were statistically significant (p <.05). SMT reduced the frequency of stuttering by about half. Beyond clinic improvement was essentially the same as within clinic improvement. Severity, as measured by the type of observed stuttering, was reduced 46%, and adverse reactions to the stuttering by 41%. Two of the six children (ST and AC) did not require any other type of treatment after SMT; the other four received Extended Length of Utterance treatment (Ingham, 1993). All but one of these children were essentially stutter-free (<1% SS) 2 years after treatment.

Speaking rate increased from 188.2 words per minute pre-SMT to 195.5 words per minute post-SMT; this change was not statistically significant. Naturalness ratings decreased (improved) significantly ($F_{[1,6]}$ = 7.4; p <.04) from 5.42 to 4.75. This decrease was about half of that needed to be within acceptable

Table 7–3. Characteristics of six children selected for speech motor training.

Subject	Sex	Age	Age at Onset	Months Postonset	Ethnic Group	Stuttering Score	Predicted Percentile
MC	m	60	40	20	EA	26	66
ST	f	49	24	25	EA	18	24
KM	m	70	28	42	HA	22	50
AW	f	77	39	38	EA	18	24
AC	f	76	47	29	EA	19	40
GS	m	62	35	27	JA	29	78
Means		65.7	35.5	30.2		24.7	47.0

Table 7–4. Stuttering frequency and severity changes associated with speech motor training.

Subject	Measures	Baseline	Withdrawal	Difference	% Difference
MC	%SS, clinic	9.01	2.59	6.42	71.3
	%SS, bynd. cl	9.51	1.86	7.65	80.4
	SPI, React.	10	5	5	50.0
	SPI, St. type	9	2	7	77.8
	SPI, total	26	10	16	61.54
ST	%SS, clinic	8.06	2.06	6.00	74.4
	%SS, bynd. cl	9.30	1.98	7.02	75.5
	SPI, React	2.0	2.0	0.00	0.0
	SPI, St. type	9	4	5	55.6
	SPI, total	18	11	7	38.9
KM	%SS, clinic	5.49	4.59	90	16.4
	%SS, bynd. cl	10.20	5.34	4.86	47.6
	SPI, React	8	6	2	25.0
	SPI, St. type	7	5	2	28.6
	SPI, total	22	17	5	22.7
AW	%SS, clinic	7.51	4.45	3.06	40.7
	%SS, bynd. cl	7.97	4.03	3.94	49.4
	SPI, React	9	8	1	11.1
	SPI, St. type	19	13	6	31.6
	SPI, total	19	13	6	31.6
AC	%SS, clinic	4.5	1.34	3.16	70.2
	%SS, bynd. cl	2.97	1.4	1.57	52.9
	SPI, React	7	1	6	85.7
	SPI, St. type	6	1	5	83.3
	SPI, total	18	5	13	72.2
GS	%SS, clinic	11.63	8.50	3.13	26.9
	%SS, bynd. cl	15.35	13.95	1.40	9.1
	SPI, React	8	4	4	50.0
	SPI, St. type	13	9	4	30.8
	SPI, total	29	21	8	27.6
Group	%SS, clinic	7.70	3.92	3.78	49.1
	%SS, bynd. cl	9.22	4.75	4.47	48.5
	SPI, React	7.33	4.33	3.00	40.9
	SPI, St. type	10.5	5.67	4.83	46.0
	SPI, total	24.67	15.00	9.67	39.0

Note: Reactions and stuttering type from *Stuttering Prediction Instrument* (Riley, 1981). Reactions include frustration, physical struggle, teasing, word avoidance, etc. Stuttering types include number and severity of part-word repetition, durations of prolongations, and tense pauses.

"norms" and was in keeping with the amount of reduction in stuttering.

Changes in Speech Motor Production

SMT is purported to affect stuttering by changing some motor planning aspects of speech production. That is, changes in speech motor planning appear related to stuttering reduction. Work in progress by Riley and Ingham (1998) suggests that following SMT children exhibit vowel durations about 37% longer and stop gap durations about 28% shorter than they did before treatment. Some other investigators have reported similar acoustic duration effects using other treatments. For examples see Mallard and Westbrook (1985); Metz, Samar, and Sacco (1983); and Robb, Lybolt, and Price (1985).

SUMMARY

- SMT developed from a theoretical framework that emphasizes the motor planning, feed-forward aspects of speech production.
- This SMT approach is justified by the evidence that children who stutter exhibit reduced functioning or integration of certain speech motor control subsystems.
- This chapter describes the fourth version of SMT, formerly called oral motor training.
- The clinical skills such as recognizing voicing errors, airflow breaks, sequencing errors, and inappropriate rate are readily learned by clinicians. Clinicians can also understand and practice the general principles of training at a slow rate and by modeling rather than explanation.
- The program employs 14 levels; difficulty is increased by adding to the number of syllables in the training set (from 1 to 2 to 3), increasing the number of unvoiced consonants in the set (from 0 to 1 to 2), and changing the shape of the set (CV to VCV to VCCV). Some sample sets are Level 1, /mou/; Level 6, /a vu/; Level 10, /næ za mi/; Level 14, /si u ve mad/.

- By using methods that require motor performance without cognitive self-monitoring, SMT avoids the problems associated with awareness of rate or manner of speaking. Naturalness is improved as stuttering is reduced.
- Stuttering frequency has been reduced an average of 49% within and beyond the clinic, and severity reduced 46%. About half of the children aged 5 years and under did not require direct stuttering modification following SMT.
- Speech motor production characteristics were changed in a manner similar to other reported changes following treatment, that is, vowels were significantly lengthened, and silence (stop gap) between vowels was significantly shortened.
- Changes in speech motor production may contribute to long-term maintenance of treatment gains because, as with learning to ride a bike, overlearned motor skills tend to remain stable.

Acknowledgments

The research examining the efficacy of SMT was supported in part by the National Institute of Health, NIDCD, Research Grant DC01100. We want to thank the dedicated clinicians who helped operationalize and refine methods to improve motor aspects of syllable production in children. Our deepest appreciation goes to Suzanne McCormick for her 17 years of clinical application and input into the development of speech motor treatment programs.

REFERENCES

Adams, M. R. (1987). Voice onsets and segment durations of normal speakers and beginning stutterers. *Journal of Fluency Disorders, 12,* 133–139.

Agnello, J., Wingate, M., & Wendell, M. (1974). *Voice onset and voice termination times of children and adult stutterers.* Paper presented at annual convention of the Acoustic Society of America, St. Louis, MO.

Bishop, J. H., Williams, H. G., & Cooper, W. A. (1991a). Age and task complexity variables in motor performances of stuttering and nonstuttering children. *Journal of Fluency Disorders, 16,* 207–217.

Bishop, J. H., Williams, H. G., & Cooper, W. A. (1991b). Age and task complexity variables in motor performance of children with articulation-disordered, stuttering, and normal speech. *Journal of Fluency Disorders, 16,* 219–228.

Borden, G. J., Harris, K. S., & Raphael, L. J. (1994). *Speech science primer: Physiology, acoustics, and perception of speech* (3rd ed.). Baltimore: Williams and Wilkins.

Cross, D., & Luper, H. (1979). Voice reaction time of stuttering and non-stuttering children and adults. *Journal of Fluency Disorders, 4,* 59–77.

Cross, D., & Luper, H. (1983). Relation between finger reaction time and voice reaction time in stuttering and nonstuttering children and adults. *Journal of Speech and Hearing Research, 26,* 356–361.

Cullinan, W., & Springer, M. (1980). Voice initiation and termination times in stuttering and nonstuttering children. *Journal of Speech and Hearing Research, 23,* 344–360.

De Nil, L. F., & Brutten, G. J. (1991). Voice onset times of stuttering and nonstuttering children: The influence of externally and linguistically imposed time pressure. *Journal of Fluency Disorders, 16,* 143–158.

Goldberg, G. (1985). Supplementary motor area structure and function: Review and hypotheses. *The Behavior and Brain Sciences, 8,* 567–616.

Healey, E. C., & Adams, M. R. (1981). Speech timing skills of normally fluent and stuttering children and adults. *Journal of Fluency Disorders, 6,* 233–246.

Howell, P., Sackin, S., & Rustin, L. (1995). Comparison of speech motor development in stutterers and fluent speakers between 7 and 12 years old. *Journal of Fluency Disorders, 20,* 243–255.

Ingham, J. C., & Riley, G. (1998). Guidelines for documentation of treatment efficacy for young children who stutter. *Journal of Speech, Language, and Hearing Research, 41,* 753–770.

Kent, R. D., & Minifie, F. D. (1977). Coarticulation in recent speech production models. *Journal of Phonetics, 5,* 115–135.

Kloth, S. A. M., Janssen, P., Kraaimaat, F. W., & Brutten, G. J. (1995). Speech-motor and linguistic skills of young stutterers prior to onset. *Journal of Fluency Disorders, 20,* 157–170.

Lashley, K. S. (1951). The problem of serial order in behavior. In L. A. Jeffress (Ed.), *Cerebral mechanisms in behavior: The Hixon symposium.* New York: John Wiley.

Lenneberg, E. H. (1967). *Biological foundations of language.* New York: John Wiley.

Liberman, A. M., Cooper, F. S., Shankweiler, D. P., & Studdert-Kennedy, M. (1967). Perception of the speech code. *Psychological Review, 74,* 431–461.

Liss, J. M., & Weismer, G. (1992). Qualitative acoustic analysis in the study of motor speech disorders. *Journal of Acoustical Society of America, 92,* 2984–2987.

MacNeilage, P. (1970). Motor control of serial ordering of speech. *Psychological Review, 77,* 182–196.

Mallard, A. R., & Westbrook, J. B. (1985). Vowel duration in stutterers participating in Precision Fluency Shaping. *Journal of Fluency Disorders, 10,* 221–228.

Maske-Cash, W. S., & Curlee, R. F. (1995). Effect of utterance length and meaningfulness on the speech initiation times of children who stutter and children who do not stutter. *Journal of Speech and Hearing Research, 38,* 18–25.

McDonald, E. (1964). *Articulation testing and treatment: A sensory-motor approach.* Pittsburgh, PA: Stanwix House.

McKnight, R., & Cullinan, W. (1987). Subgroups of stuttering children: Speech and voice reaction times, segmental durations, and naming latencies. *Journal of Fluency Disorders, 12,* 217–233.

Metz, D. E., Samar, V. C., & Sacco, P. R. (1983). Acoustic analysis of stutterers' fluent speech before and after therapy. *Journal of Speech and Hearing Research, 26,* 531–536.

Murphy, M., & Baumgartner, J. M. (1981). Voice initiation and termination time in stuttering and nonstuttering children. *Journal of Fluency Disorders, 6,* 257–264.

Riley, G. (1981). *Stuttering Prediction Instrument for young children.* Austin, TX: Pro-Ed.

Riley, G., & Ingham, J. C. (1998). *Acoustic duration changes associated with two types of treatment for children who stutter.* In review.

Riley, G., & Riley, J. (1985). *Oral motor assessment and treatment: Improving syllable production.* Austin, TX: Pro-Ed.

Riley, G., & Riley, J. (1986). Oral motor discoordination among children who stutter. *Journal of Fluency Disorders, 11,* 334–344.

Riley, G., & Riley, J. (1991). Treatment implications of oral motor discoordination. In H. F. M. Peters, W. Hulstijn, & C. W. Starkweather (Eds.), *Speech motor control and stuttering* (pp. 471–476). Amsterdam: Elsevier Science Publishers.

Robb, M., Lybolt, J., & Price, H. (1985). Acoustic measures of stutterers' speech following an intensive therapy program. *Journal of Fluency Disorders, 10,* 269–279.

Sharf, D. J., & Ohde, R. N. (1981). Physiologic, acoustic and perceptual aspects of coarticulation: Implications for the remediation of articulatory disorders. In N. J. Lass (Ed.), *Speech and language: Advances in basic research and practice* (Vol. 5, pp. 153–247). New York: Academic Press.

Stetson, R. (1951). Motor phonetics. Amsterdam: North-Holland. Sussman, H. M., Hoemeke, K., & McCaffrey, H. A. (1992). Locus equations as an index of coarticulation for place of articulation distinctions in children. *Journal of Speech and Hearing Research, 35,* 769–781.

Sussman, H.M., Hoemeke, K., & McCaffrey, H.A. (1992). Locus equations as an index of coarticulation for place of articulation distinctions in children. *Journal of Speech and Hearing Research, 35,* 769–781.

Till, J., Reich, A., Dickey, S., & Seiber, J. (1983). Phonatory and manual reaction times of stuttering and nonstuttering children. *Journal of Speech and Hearing Research, 26,* 171–180.

Wall, M. J., Starkweather, C. W., & Harris, K. S. (1981). The influence of voicing adjustments on the location of stuttering in the spontaneous speech of young child stutterers. *Journal of Fluency Disorders, 6,* 299–310.

Weismer, G., Kent, R. D., Hodge, M., & Martin, R. (1988). The acoustic signature for intelligibility test words. *Journal of Acoustical Society of America, 84,* 1281–1291.

Williams, H. G., & Bishop, J. H. (1992). Speed and consistency of manual movements of stutterers, articulation disordered children and children with normal speech. *Journal of Fluency Disorders, 17,* 191–203.

Zebrowski, P., Conture, E., & Cudahy, E. (1985). Acoustic analysis of young stutterers' fluency. *Journal of Fluency Disorders, 10,* 173–192.

The Fluency Rules Program

CHARLES M. RUNYAN
SARA ELIZABETH RUNYAN

INTRODUCTION

The Fluency Rules Program (FRP) was conceived and designed to provide therapeutic direction to help preschool and early grade-school stutterers acquire fluent speech. Prior to 1986, the date of the first publication of the FRP, limited therapeutic material was available for use with young stutterers. Not surprisingly, in 1976, our first year of university teaching, the first question asked by public school speech-language pathologists was, "How do we work with young stutterers?" From 1976 until 1981 when the FRP was developed and initially implemented, we evaluated and treated young stutterers both in the University Clinic and as consultants to elementary schools in the Shenandoah Valley of Virginia. The focus of our initial therapeutic efforts was to take well accepted, physiologically based therapy principles used with adult stutterers and, with modifications, apply them to children. These beginning therapy attempts to teach children the association between physiology and fluency were reasonably successful and were labeled "rules of good speech." By 1981, these clinical techniques were known as Fluency Rules.

Originally there were 10 rules designed to teach children to speak fluently and sound natural. Our greatest therapeutic challenge during this developmental stage was the "translation" of anatomical and physiological concepts into language young children could comprehend and use. However, with continued clinical effort and expanded therapy experience with young stutterers, the number of rules was reduced and the instructions for them were simplified. Based on these clinical experiences the effectiveness and utility of each rule was evaluated; as a result some rules remained unchanged, some were eliminated, and others were modified until the final seven rules of the FRP were established.

Initially, all Fluency Rules with associated instructions were presented to every young stutterer. During this developmental phase, the child was required to practice all the fluency rules using therapeutic drill work. It soon became apparent that this rather complex and intense procedure was neither time efficient nor therapeutically effective for delivering clinical services. Teaching all the rules and explaining the principles associated with each rule consumed significant therapy time and, more importantly, required the speech-language pathologist to teach skills that the children frequently possessed. In other words, children did not come to therapy breaking all the fluency rules. Therefore, when the FRP was published in 1986 (Runyan & Runyan, 1986), the treatment program consisted of seven fluency rules with therapy instructions and directions to address only rules that the child had not mastered. The initial treatment results were positive, and subsequent implementation of the FRP has not changed the number of rules; application of the rules has significantly altered in a continued effort to maximize treatment results.

With daily use of the FRP, we became aware that the rules were being presented in a specific sequence rather than all at one time. This emerging method of presentation was especially true for preschool and special population children (e.g., learning disabled, autistic, cerebral palsied). This new order of presentation became the basis for FRP-R published in 1995 (Runyan & Runyan, 1993). The revised FRP procedure provided a structure and order for the presentation of the rules. The rules that had consistently been presented first to every child became the Universal Rules. The next two rules, the Primary Rules, were physiologically based rules, which were used with children who exhibited breathing and laryngeal problems associated with instances of stuttering. Finally, Secondary Rules were used only when secondary behaviors were a component of the stuttering blocks.

THE PROGRAM

The remainder of this chapter describes the individual Fluency Rules and how they are applied. Particular emphasis is given to program implementation and therapy techniques that have been effective with preschool stutterers, early grade-school stutterers, and special population stutterers.

Universal Rules

There are two Universal Rules: "Speak Slowly" and "Say a Word One Time." These two rules are usually the only rules necessary to treat very young stutterers. However, for young stutterers who also demonstrate prolongations, the Secondary Rule, "Say it Short," is included as a Universal Rule. The intent of Universal Rules is to provide basic instructions to assist the child in producing fluent speech.

Rule 1: Speak Slowly (Turtle Speech)

This rule is presented first to encourage a reduced rate of speech production. Reduction in rate may provide additional time for the development of self-monitoring skills, which the child can use to acquire and develop physiologic skills necessary for fluent speech production. Although this rule has always been labeled "speak slowly" or "turtle speech," the intent was never to encourage children to produce abnormally slow speech or to say words one at a time in a rhythmic pattern. In fact, in our clinical experience young children acquiring linguistic competency are not concerned with the rate of speech production. The message, not speech rate, is important to the child, and attempts to manipulate the rate of speech to an abnormally slow rate have not been therapeutically beneficial. During early developmental stages of the FRP-R, attempts were made to have children increase the length of their fluent speech by producing one word, then two words, then three words, and so on using a slow rate of speech. These attempts met significant therapeutic resistance from both the child and the parents because the speech pattern sounded abnormal, and both were reluctant to use this speech pattern outside the clinic.

As we continued to use the Speak Slowly Rule clinically, an unexpected benefit associated with this rule became apparent. Therapy data repeatedly revealed the frequency of stuttering decreasing while speech rate remained virtually unchanged. After repeated observations, clinicians and parents were interviewed and we concluded that the reduction in the frequency of stuttering may be due to a general calming effect. This calming effect appeared to be a by-product of the modeled slow rate of speech encouraged by this Universal Rule in the therapy sessions and home environment.

In previous publications, use of symbolic material (e.g., turtles and snails) was suggested to teach the concept of slow speech rate, by contrasting "slow" symbolic material with "fast" symbolic material (e.g., racehorses). Illustrating the importance of slow and careful speech by using an analogy of walking slowly and carefully, not rapidly and carelessly, has been an effective technique. A physical demonstration, accompanied by a verbal description, gives the therapist an opportunity to explain that fast walking creates slips and falls (we act these out by falling on the floor!), while slower walking is easy and without consequence. Likewise, if speech is too rapid then words may be "tripped over" and repeated, but with a slow rate speech is smooth and flowing.

Modeling a slow rate of speech production has also been successfully used with very young beginning stutterers. Not only is the slow rate of speech modeled in the clinical setting, but parents also are encouraged to use this technique at home. Parents are instructed to model the slow rate of speech but cautioned not to repeatedly remind the child to talk slower. If followed correctly, this procedure allows the parents to become active participants in the therapy process, providing additional therapy support outside the clinic setting.

As effective as the previous therapy techniques have been, the most successful technique to teach slow rate was the addition of a nonverbal cue to slow down. To accomplish this the clinician moves a hand using an up-and-down motion, the traditional hand signal to slow down. This visual cue can be used whenever the child increases speech rate above the therapy target rate. With continued use, the therapeutic intent of the hand signal quickly becomes meaningful, and it can then be effectively used without verbal instruction to teach the concept of slowing down. An added benefit is that this technique requires minimal therapy time to teach, because the hand signal to slow down is easily and widely understood.

Rule 2: Say a Word One Time

This rule is the foundation of the FRP when treating very young children. Obviously, part-word and whole-word repetitions are the speech characteristics typically exhibited by young disfluent children. A technique to control these repetitions must be a vital component of any treatment program designed for this population. To use this rule effectively, children must understand the concept of one, once, or one time. To teach this concept, sequential materials such as days of the week or months of the year, letters of the alphabet, and numbers in a row have been helpful. An explanation is provided that each word is unique and does not need to be said more than one time. Then the child and the therapist repeat one of the series of words in unison. To demonstrate the concept further in an animated fashion, the therapist selects one word from the series and repeats this word 20 times (e.g., One, two, two, two [20×]) while bouncing up and down with the production of each number. This redundancy and animated physical activity captures the child's attention and allows the therapist to ask, "Did I need to say the word more than one time for you to understand it?" The response has always been "no." This dialog helps the child understand the importance of "being careful about what we say and listening to make sure we say each word only one time."

To ensure the success of this rule and the development of self-monitoring skills necessary for therapeutic progress, the child is encouraged to identify repeated words produced by the therapist. During this phase of therapy, the clinician intentionally and frequently repeats words and part words and the child is encouraged to signal when these repetitions occur. Therapy session data are recorded first on how correctly and later on how rapidly the child identifies these instances of repetitions. When clinician-generated repetitions are identified correctly every time, the child is asked if we can help identify repeated words in her or his speech. Therapy continues with the both the therapist and the child identifying repetitions in each other's speech. This procedure takes the format of a game with each participant trying to "catch" the other repeating a word. As the child becomes more fluent and there are fewer opportunities for repetitions, to keep awareness high, the clinician should produce increasingly more repetitions so that the intent of therapy is not lost. As a final step, the focus of therapy is turned to the child's speech by encouraging the child to identify when the repetitions occur in his or her own speech and on which word. Again this technique can be turned into a game, with the clinician and the child competing to determine who can identify the child's repetition first.

Two additional therapy techniques have proven effective in teaching this Universal Rule. The first technique called "Old Ears" can be used with either Universal Rule. With a great deal of animation (e.g., pulling down on our sagging ear) the child is shown our "Very Old Ears," and we explain that when people repeat words "it really hurts our old ears." Therefore, "please don't repeat words, instead say just one word at a time and this will be gentle to our old ears." If the child repeats a word again, we grab our "old ears," and with a great deal of exaggeration, say and demonstrate (e.g., falling down and rolling on the floor) how painful these repetitions are to our ears. Of course, this is done in a humorous fashion, so the child is not frightened but does understand the importance of saying a word one time. The second technique, taught at the beginning of this Universal Rule, is to have the child raise an index finger when he hears the therapist repeat a word or sound. We explain that this signal will remind the therapist to say each word once. Of course, when the focus of therapy turns to the child's speech, the therapist uses the same reminder. This raised index finger signal has the added benefit of not interrupting the talker during a conversational turn. A further benefit is that this technique can be used with minimal effort at home and gives the parents the opportunity for an expanded role in the therapeutic process. Our most dramatic therapy success occurred when a child spontaneously used this signaling technique at home during dinner to indicate that a parent had repeated a word. Obviously, the child understood the concept of saying a word one time, and therapy was successfully concluded shortly after this event occurred.

Secondary Rule (Third Universal Rule)

The intent of this rule is to assist the stutterer therapeutically to eliminate prolongations. For maximum results this rule must be applied immediately following every instance of a prolongation.

Rule Three: Say it Short

This rule becomes a Universal Rule for very young stutterers who exhibit prolongations. When needed, the most effective therapy technique is another hand signal. The hand signal is the well-known signal for short, which is placing the thumb and forefinger close together. Because this nonverbal hand signal is so well known, therapy time needed to teach this concept has been minimal.

Primary Rules

The Primary Rules are used to treat aspects of stuttering that appear to be physiologically based. Children treated using the

Primary Rules have demonstrated abnormal breathing patterns or laryngeal activity (during their stuttering blocks). These physiological behaviors usually are not manifested in the speech of preschoolers. However, the Primary Rules have been used with children as young as second grade. When use of the Primary Rules is necessary, based on the diagnosis or clinical observation, they are taught as a package. In other words, if a child experiences difficulty with speech breathing or laryngeal tension, then an explanation of speech production incorporating both primary rules is undertaken.

Rule Four: Use Speech Breathing

To explain speech breathing, a breath curve is drawn on paper or a chalkboard, using a steep slope upward to indicate rapid inspiration and a gradual downward slope for slow exhalation. Then this drawing is related to what occurs physiologically when the child breathes. To relate the drawing in a tactile manner to breathing, the child's hand is placed just below the sternum with the clinician's hand on top, so "the rise and fall" of the chest wall can be felt. After the child comprehends the relationship of chest wall movements and breathing, this breathing pattern is related to speech production. To do so, an "X" is placed on the down slope just after the peak on the breathing curve where inhalation ends and exhalation begins. The child is told that this "X" is the point during exhalation at which to start speech. With hands properly positioned and the breath curve drawing set up for easy viewing, the child is instructed to trace the breath curve with a finger while feeling the corresponding movements of the chest wall. Once this procedure has been practiced and understood, speech is introduced using the designated "X." The first speaking tasks include the sequential material used during practice of the Universal Rules (i.e., counting, days of the week, etc.). Following this activity short simple phrases are repeated, none of which begins with a sound associated with stuttering. During these drill activities, we explain and demonstrate that we speak on exhalation, and that "air carries the words out." To teach this concept, again in a humorous fashion, we demonstrate with exaggerated effort that speech cannot be produced when we hold our breath.

Rule Five: Start Mr. Voice Box Running Smoothly/Gently

For the young stutterer this rule is infrequently used. If needed, we incorporate gentle onset of voicing with speech breathing by instructing the child to exhale slowly, feeling the air as it "comes up the throat," and at the designated "X" to start to hum gently. This activity is followed by having the child repeat phrases with the initial word beginning with /m/. On occasion, depending on the child's age and comprehension ability, an awareness technique is needed to explain that "Mr. Voice Box lives in the neck." To demonstrate this point, we phonate or hum while shaking our neck vigorously with our hand and hear the funny sound this activity causes, thus proving that Mr. Voice Box lives in our neck.

Program Implementation

The FRP is implemented in the following manner.

1. Determine the Rules That Are Broken

For the very young stutterer, the usual area for therapeutic intervention is the elimination of repetitions and, on occasion, prolongations. Therefore, for all young stutterers, the Universal Rules Speak Slowly and Say A Word One Time are used, with Rule 3: Say it Short included when prolonged speech is a concern.

2. Teach the Necessary Concepts

The prerequisite concepts (e.g., slow, one time, short) for understanding each Fluency Rule are taught. The techniques described following each Fluency Rule assist in teaching these concepts.

3. Develop the Child's Self-Monitoring Skills

When the therapist is confident that the child comprehends the concepts associated with the rules, then the child's awareness of when to apply the rules has begun. As previously stated, this process starts when the child "catches" the clinician violating the rules. At first, the therapist supplies the speech examples (i.e., frequent examples of breaking the rules), allowing the child to practice monitoring the therapist's conversational speech. When the child has identified the broken rule, the therapist repeats the phrase observing the rule, and thanks the child for helping. After a short period (two to three therapy sessions), the child usually can quickly identify with 100% accuracy the broken rule(s) in the therapist's speech. Teaching the child to self-monitor, the next treatment phase, is accomplished by again thanking the child for helping us with our speech and asking if we can help with his or her speech if we hear a rule broken. At first, we encourage the child to tell us what "word" broke the rule and to "say it the better way." Therapy continues with the child and the therapist identifying broken rules in each other's speech.

4. Therapeutic Practice Using the Rules

The most important clinical principle for young children is that therapy must be fun. When therapy is fun, learning becomes a natural part of the therapy process. Thus, the format of therapy for young stutterers is play. Most therapy sessions are 60 minutes long and take place on the floor playing with age-appropriate games and toys. The child is allowed to direct the course of the play. If the child throws toys, screams, or attempts other disruptive behaviors, rules for play in the clinical setting are quickly established. The most effective procedure in our practice is that play time is stopped when disruptive behavior occurs, and the child and the therapist sit at "the therapy table" and "say words fluently" in a very structured drill manner. This drill activity is obviously not as much fun as playing on the floor, and the child quickly changes the disruptive behavior. During play sessions, the therapist and the child identify instances when the Fluency Rules are not used. Currently we conduct almost all of our therapeutic intervention using the hand signals described throughout the chapter. By using the FRP-R in this manner, the therapist can correct or point out broken rules without interrupting the child's speech or having the child lose a conversational turn. Entire treatment sessions using only the nonverbal cues occur frequently, particularly close to the termination of therapy. During this later stage of therapy the child does not have to correct the disfluent words.

5. Carryover to the Home and/or Classroom

The use of nonverbal cues has made transition of the Fluency Rules and fluent speech to environments outside the clinic easier and more productive. Both teachers and parents can use the same hand signals, thus keeping awareness of the rules at a high level. The obvious benefit for everyone is consistency. The hand signals can be used easily in almost any environment without direct verbal intervention. Eliminating the direct verbal confrontation reduces conflicts and keeps the child more receptive to additional therapeutic directions. The ability of parents and teachers to employ these nonverbal reminders leads to more rapid generalization of fluent speech outside the speech clinic.

Stickers (we use elephants because elephants never forget!) or other visual reminders strategically placed in the classroom and home also have been effective in keeping the child aware of the Fluency Rules. Similarly, allowing the child to borrow a favorite toy from the clinic has proven to be an effective treatment tool for transferring the Fluency Rules and fluent speech from the clinic to the home. For stutterers in the early grades who are playing video games, we have successfully used a lending library of video games to assist in the transfer of the Fluency Rules to the home environment. These video and computer games have tremendous motivational value for this age group. To check out or borrow toys or games, the child must agree to: (a) use the Fluency Rules at home, (b) allow the parents to participate and "help us" (i.e., the therapist) by using the hand signals at home, and (c) return the toy or game the next therapy session. This procedure has increased parent involvement, and both parents and children have reported positive interactions at home without the tension usually associated with other parental reminders. The telephone has also been used as an effective reminder of the Fluency Rules in the home environment. With the parents' permission, we call the child frequently and ask about fluency, or whether they are enjoying the toy or game. After a short period and a number of phone calls, the child thinks the therapist is calling every time the phone rings and the phone acts as a reminder of the Fluency Rules.

EVALUATION OF THE PROGRAM

Previous publications (Runyan & Runyan, 1986, 1993) reported the therapeutic effectiveness of the FRP with 23 young stutterers, 6 of whom were of preschool age. Five of the six children successfully finished the treatment program with fluent speech. One subject left our geographic area shortly after therapy began, and subsequent attempts to contact the family failed. Since the second publication, five additional preschool stutterers have been treated at our practice (see Table 8–1). To date, all have completed the program with fluent, natural sounding speech. All have remained fluent based on follow-up contacts, with the possible exception of HH, whose family recently contacted our office to schedule another visit. The telephone request indicated only a mild concern, but if the reported quality of speech continued the family would call and make an appointment.

Table 8–1. Preschool subjects treated using FRP.

Subject	Age	Sex	Severity[1]	Family History[2]	Postonset
CB	3 years, 2 months	M	Moderate (20)	+	4 months
CB	5 years, 1 month	F	Moderate (23)	–	2+ years
HH	4 years, 7 months	F	Moderate (25)	–	3+ years
MP	4 years, 1 month	M	Moderate (20)	–	2+ years
RM	5 years	F	Moderate (20)	+	2+ years

[1] SSI scores in parentheses.

[2] + indicates positive family history of stuttering.

SUMMARY

- In the FRP, there are two Universal Rules, "Speak Slowly" and "Say a Word One Time."
- "Say it Short" becomes a Universal Rule for the very young stutterer who exhibits prolongations.
- The Primary Rules of the FRP treatment aspects of stuttering that appear to be physiologically based are; "Use Speech Breathing," and "Start Mr. Voice Box Running Smoothly/Gently."
- Maximum therapeutic success occurs with the FRP when both professionals and parents apply the treatment techniques consistently to a stuttering child. The FRP encourages and includes active involvement of the public school speech-language pathologist.
- The FRP program emphasizes the importance of generalization.

REFERENCES

Runyan, C. M., & Runyan, S. E. (1986). Fluency rules therapy program for young children in the public school. *Language, Speech and Hearing Services in Schools, 17,* 276–284.

Runyan, C. M., & Runyan, S. E. (1993). Therapy for school-aged stutterers: An update on the Fluency Rules Program. In R. Curlee (Ed.), *Stuttering and related disorders of fluency.* (pp. 101–114) New York: Thieme.

9

The Monterey Fluency Program

BRUCE P. RYAN

BARBARA VAN KIRK RYAN

INTRODUCTION

The Monterey Fluency Program (MFP) was developed in the late 1960s and early 1970s. It was based on learning principles, in particular, operant conditioning. The major target for people of all ages who stutter, is normally fluent speech. The MFP involves speech only, because we and others have observed that changes in attitude and anxiety often occurred after changes in fluency (e.g., Craig et al., 1996; Ingham, 1984; Ryan, 1974; Ryan & Ryan, 1983, 1995). In this chapter, our discussion focuses on preschool children (2 to 5 years of age) and the application of the MFP, with modifications, to this population.

Part of the information in this chapter about treating preschool children who stutter comes from the first author's experience in the university setting while conducting the Genesis of Stuttering Project, a 15-year cross-sectional, longitudinal, single-subject study of the development of stuttering of 50 preschool stuttering children (Ryan, 1984a, 1985a, 1990, 1992, 1993, 1998a; Ryan & Marsh, 1989). Part of the information comes from the second author's experiences with conducting the MFP with preschool children in the public school setting.

THE PROGRAM

The MFP is based on the three major components of programmed instruction and operant conditioning: (a) overt responses (stuttering and fluent speech), (b) small steps or successive approximation (e.g., one fluent word, two fluent words, etc.), and (c) immediate consequences (e.g., positive, "Good," for fluent utterances and corrective feedback or punishment, "Stop, speak fluently," for stutterings). Tokens with backup reinforcers (e.g., toys) are also used with children. Additional components are the requirements of some reasonable duration of performance (e.g., a criterion of 10 consecutive correct or fluent words) and continuous on-line (real time) collection of data to achieve the target of normally fluent speech. These procedures make the MFP amenable to clinical trials of efficacy (Ingham & Riley, 1998).

Ryan (1974) observed that clients referred to his clinic for stuttering were above 3 stuttered words per minute (SW/M). Craven and Ryan (1985) observed that, although almost all normally fluent speakers *stutter*, if one considers whole- and part-word repetitions as stuttered words, normally fluent speakers demonstrate less than 3 SW/M. Further, Ryan (1998c) observed that normally fluent preschool children performed the same as the children and adults in Craven and Ryan's earlier study (1985). Hence, we have used the criterion of 3 SW/M, along with other criteria, as the cutoff between those who are considered to stutter and those who are not. However, as can be noted in most of our past research (e.g., Ryan & Ryan, 1983, 1995), our within-program criterion has been less than 0.5 SW/M and our stuttering clients have generally been under 1 SW/M immediately post-treatment and at follow-up (Ryan, 1981). Of course, speaking rate is also taken into consideration, and we have expected and observed that most clients do speak more rapidly post-treatment due to the elimination of stuttering.

There are three phases of treatment: establishment (within-clinic fluency), transfer (out-of-clinic fluency), and maintenance (fluency within and out of the clinic over time) (Ryan, 1974). The MFP is a performance-driven clinical treatment with a built-in data collection system. A number of clinicians in several countries have been trained to carry out the program (Rustin, Ryan, & Ryan, 1987; Ryan, 1985c; Ryan & Ryan, 1994). We and others have used these procedures with children and adults for the past 27 years (Rustin, Ryan, & Ryan, 1987; Ryan, 1985b, 1985c, 1998c; Ryan & Ryan, 1983, 1994, 1995, 1998).

The MFP, designed to develop speech fluency for children and adults, initiated by Ryan and Van Kirk (1971), continued to be revised until it reached its final form in Ryan and Van Kirk (1978). An outline of the full program, including testing for older children and adults, is presented first so that the revisions for preschool children can be evaluated in the context of knowledge of the full program.

Two tests are built into the program, because we adhered to the instructional programming principle of *test-teach-test* (Pipe, 1966). First, the Fluency Interview, which is composed of 10 speaking tasks ranging from automatic (e.g., counting) to conversational speech with strangers, and second, a Criterion Test (5 minutes each of reading, monologue, and conversation) are administered. These two tests serve to determine the level of pre-treatment stuttering and as post-tests to determine improvement and effectiveness of the treatment program at various stages.

Following the administration of these two tests, the client progresses through a speech fluency program which contains steps in three phases: establishment, transfer, and maintenance. A flow chart with all the procedures and decisions to be made is shown in Ryan (1974, p. 66, Figure 11). An outline of the MFP procedures for older children and adults with times of tasks is:

- Fluency Interview composed of 11 speaking tasks (15 min).
- Criterion Test composed of reading (5 min), monologue (5 min), and conversation (5 min).
- If client demonstrates stuttering rate above 3 SW/M on either test, go on to Establishment Program.
- Establishment program of Gradual Increase in Length and Complexity of Utterance (GILCU) of 54 steps (18 in reading, 18 in monologue, and 18 in conversation), which start with the client reading one word fluently and end with the client conversing fluently for 5 min. Home practice after reading, monologue, and conversation completed.

or
(for older clients with more severe stuttering)

- Establishment program of Delayed Auditory Feedback (DAF) (prolongation) of 26 steps (5 in learning prolonged speech, 7 in reading, 7 in monologue, and 7 in conversation), which start with the client speaking in a slow, prolonged manner (40 words per min) for a sentence and end with the client conversing for 5 min normally fluently at a normal speaking rate. Home practice after reading, monologue, and conversation completed.

- Both GILCU and DAF (prolongation) clients progress to the next test.
- Another Criterion Test after completing either DAF (prolongation) or GILCU, and if client is below 0.5 SW/M, go on to Transfer program; if not, recycle Establishment program.
- Transfer program of age-appropriate steps (maximum of 54 steps, e.g., speak with audience of 1–3 people, telephone, school or work).
- Another Criterion Test after Transfer program; if below 0.5 SW/M, progress to Maintenance; if not, recycle parts of the Establishment and Transfer programs.
- Maintenance program (5 recheck steps gradually faded over a 2-year period).
- Follow-up 1 or more years after completion of last program step or test.[1]

The design of the MFP permitted it to meet the efficacy criterion of clear description of the procedure. The MFP clinician's manual, which describes these procedures in some detail, is 72 double spaced pages in length. This book provides a detailed "script" in outline form for the clinician to follow while carrying out the program after training. This detail increases the probability of accurate replication in the clinician's own site (see results of training in Ryan, 1985c). An example of the detail of the instructions from the training program is:

Tell the client to speak fluently for 2 minutes. Use a stop watch to time only the client's talking. If the client speaks fluently for 2 consecutive minutes of talk time, say "Good." If not, say "Stop" on each stuttered word, have the client stop speaking, and reset the stop watch. Keep doing this until the client can speak fluently for 2 minutes.

Data collection, using prescribed forms, is mandatory both to aid the clinician in making decisions about moving through

---

[1]Although not an official part of the original MFP, we carried out this follow-up (e.g., Ryan, 1981), and the first author did follow-up of preschool stuttering children routinely in the Genesis of Stuttering project.

the program and to demonstrate the program's effectiveness in reducing stuttering. We desired to produce a program that could be used by a variety of clinicians in a variety of settings with some training and minimal equipment. The easiest to follow and most readily available description and outline of the MFP is in Ryan (1984b).

Modifications for Preschool Children

For evaluation of preschool stuttering children, we added speech and language tests to the Fluency Interview, because these children often demonstrated articulation and language errors along with their stuttering (Ryan, 1992). To control for spontaneous recovery (see discussion in Bloodstein, 1995, pp. 112–116, and Curlee & Yairi, 1997) in the preschool population, the first author tested monthly for at least 3 months to determine the stability of the stuttering before starting treatment. If the fluency improved (SW/M decreased), the first author continued to retest until the parents reported, and the testing supported that report, that the problem was gone, then the first author did follow-up testing for several years (Ryan, 1984a, 1998b). If the problem stayed the same or became worse, the first author began treatment.

The revised MFP treatment procedures for use with preschool children who stutter are found in Table 9-1. We omitted the reading, talking on the telephone, and talking with strangers items from the Fluency Interview. Instead, we observed the mother speaking with the child for 10 min (Ryan, 1984a, 1998a). Mothers have almost always been able to evoke what appears to be normal conversation with their children when we have been occasionally unsuccessful. In the public school setting, because of time constraints, the second author also reduced the Criterion Test from 5 min of talking time to 3 min of talking time in order to complete both monologue and conversation in the same 20-min session. The first author also asked the parents to continuously rate the severity (1, mild, to 7, severe) of the child's stuttering outside the clinic setting. The mother was asked, "As of today and the past month, is your child still stuttering?" If the answer was "no," the interview proceeded to the next question. If the answer was "yes," the mother was asked, " If 1 is mild and 7 is severe, what number would you pick to describe the severity of your child's stuttering?" The first author discovered that most mothers could accurately rate their children's stuttering behavior (Takata, 1989); that is, their ratings correlated with our objective measure of SW/M. This rating provided an easily obtain-

Table 9-1. The MFP revised for preschool children: Testing, establishment, transfer, maintenance, and follow-up.

Activity	Number of Steps, Criteria, and Times
Testing	
Fluency Interview, Parent Conversation	8 speaking activities 15 min, 10 min
Criterion Test in Monologue/Conversation	3 or 5 min each
Establishment (36 steps)	
Monologue	18 steps starting with one word and ending with 5 min of fluent monologue (0 SW/M)
Practice at home in monologue	5 min monologue daily
Conversation	18 steps starting with one word and ending with 5 min of fluent conversation (0 SW/M)
Practice at home in conversation	5 min conversation daily
Testing	
Fluency Interview, Parent Conversation	8 speaking activities 15 min, 10 min
Criterion Test in Monologue/Conversation	3 or 5 min each, at less than .5 SW/M
Transfer (13 steps)	
Talk with clinician in different physical settings	5 steps starting outside the clinic room and ending in preschool classroom or clinic waiting room. 3 consecutive min of fluent speech in conversation (0 SW/M).
Talk at clinic with friends/family	3 steps starting with 1 person ending with 3 persons. 3 consecutive min of fluent speech in conversation (0 SW/M)
Talk at clinic and home with parents	5 steps starting with parent in the clinic room and siblings, relatives, and friends. 3 consecutive min of fluent speech in conversation (0 SW/M)
Testing	
Fluency Interview, Parent Conversation	8 speaking activities 15 min, 10 min
Criterion Test in Monologue/Conversation	3 or 5 min each at less than 0.5 SW/M

Table 9-1. (continued)

Activity	Number of Steps, Criteria, and Times
Maintenance (5 steps)	
	5 steps gradually fading clinic contact: 2 weeks, 1 month, 3 months, 6 months, and 12 months. 3 consecutive min of fluent speech in conversation. Recycle if above 1 SW/M
Follow-up (1 or 2 steps)	
At 1 or 2 years	
Fluency Interview, Parent Conversation	8 speaking activities 15 min, 10 min

able estimate of the child's extra-clinic stuttering pretreatment or of generalization of the new fluency observed to the child's environment. This procedure provided us with information about the representativeness of our in-clinic sample (Ryan, 1984a).

Both authors have used mainly the GILCU establishment program rather than DAF (prolonged speech) with preschool children, with the modification of employing the modes of monologue and/or conversation only, omitting the mode of reading. Occasionally, with very young children who were incapable of monologue (and there were very few), we used only conversation. Occasionally, the "maturity" of the child determined how soon he or she formally started GILCU. A child's inability to attend to the task of sitting and/or to respond to the desired requests of the MFP required the second author initially to train the child to sit and respond, using simple game playing activities. The MFP, much as described in Table 9-1, was then conducted by the second author with the child. The first author found that most preschool children who stuttered were quite talkative; in fact, this was one of the distinguishing characteristics between them and their nonstuttering controls (Ryan, 1984a).

Next, we reduced the Transfer program to three series for a total of 13 steps: different physical settings, audience increase, and home. We often omitted the home series because home practice obviated its necessity. The first author omitted the school or classroom transfer series because a number of preschoolers did not go to any school. Often, we did not need a formal transfer program at all because the younger the child, the greater the amount of spontaneous generalization (Ryan, 1971; Ryan & Ryan, 1983, 1995). The parent's rating of stuttering severity outside the clinic served to help determine whether or not to do transfer. If the parents reported continued stuttering outside the clinic setting, we would institute the Transfer program.

The Maintenance program was also reduced with preschool children. Follow-up, although not part of the original MFP, was commonly done by the first author to obtain clinical research information about long-term results. Follow-up was often easily or naturally available in the public school setting simply by the circumstance of being there over time, and the second author did follow-up when circumstances permitted.

Data Collection

An important characteristic of the MFP is the continuous collection of objective SW/M data, and for preschool children, parent ratings of severity of stuttering (Ryan, 1984a; Takata, 1989), and, occasionally, speaking rate data. In our experience and research we have observed that preschool children have a natural tendency to achieve normal speaking rates without clinical attention, which may be explained by their sensitivity to parent or clinician models (Jones & Ryan, 1998; Ryan, 1984a, 1990, 1998a, 1998c; Wood & Ryan, in press).

Stuttering Rate

Stuttering is the main dependent variable or behavior to be modified when working with preschoolers. In our opinion and experience, anxiety and attitude problems do not play much of a role in this young population (Ryan, 1984a, 1985a, 1990, 1993, Ryan & Marsh, 1989). We focus almost entirely on the production of fluent speech with the child and information for the parent along with home practice.

We use a stuttering identification procedure of whole-word repetitions, part-word repetitions, prolongation, and struggle, after Johnson (1961) as modified by Ryan (1974) and discussed recently by Silverman (1995). The inclusion of whole- and part-word repetitions as stuttered words means that we will also find these behaviors both at some level post-treatment in the speech of our clients and in the speech of normally fluent speakers (Craven & Ryan, 1985). We do not discriminate between single and multiple whole- or part-word repetitions. We have a 90-min training program on audiotape to teach the identification of stuttered words, which we have used with over 500 clinicians and clients around the world (Ryan, 1985c; Ryan & Ryan, 1994, 1998; Ryan & Van Kirk, 1973).

We count stuttered words with a hand counter, and measure talking time (client's talking only) with a stopwatch. We then compute stuttered words per minute (SW/M), by dividing the number of stuttered words by the talking time of the client. For example, 20 stutters in 2 min of talking equals 10 SW/M (20/2). The major value of this metric is its consistency despite variation in sample size (e.g., 2 stuttered words in 1 min is comparable to 20 stuttered words in 10 min, as both yield 2 SW/M). The metrics of percentages of stuttered words or syllables require the clinician to count words or syllables. The metric of SW/M correlates very highly with percent stuttering (.91; Ryan & Ryan, 1995, p. 68) and moderately with rating scales of severity (mean of six correlation coefficients = .51; Takata, 1989). We have continued to use the measure SW/M rather than change to stuttered syllables per minute (SS/M) because we have not seen the necessity. Our data (Ryan, 1984a, 1985a, 1990, 1992, 1993; Ryan & Marsh, 1989) have suggested no statistically significant or clinical difference between SW/M and SS/M, and preschool children seldom stutter on more than one syllable in a word or use multiple syllabic words longer than two syllables. We have continued to use this simple measure because it is easy to carry a small stopwatch and hand counter almost anywhere to collect SW/M and do the simple arithmetic to convert total stutterings divided by time to SW/M.

Speaking Rate

We have also counted both words and syllables and determined words spoken or read per minute (WS/M) (Ryan, 1974; Ryan & Ryan, 1983, 1995) and syllables spoken per minute (SPM) (Ryan, 1992). These data were of less importance to us than SW/M and are much more time-consuming to collect. We have collected these data in our research mostly to support the notion that subjects were speaking normally, without stuttering, at normal speaking rates (e.g., Ryan & Ryan, 1995).

As a clinician-researcher, the first author routinely obtained speaking rate measures of all interactions with preschool children who stutter (Ryan, 1984). The first author (Jones & Ryan,

1998; Ryan, 1998a; Wood & Ryan, in press) has used the computer-aided Stuttering Treatment Rating Recorder (STRR) (Fowler & Ingham, 1986; and as used in, e.g., Onslow, Adams, & Ingham, 1992) to obtain continuous measures of speaking rate (along with stuttering rate). This equipment permits the user to press one button for a fluent syllable or word and one for a stuttered syllable or word. The computer then computes SPM. As a clinician who carried a case load of 75 clients per week (only a few of whom were children who stuttered), the second author found such continuous measurement time consuming and unnecessary. Our clinical compromise has been to do speaking rate analysis only during pre- and postcriterion tests (Ryan & Van Kirk, 1971, 1974a, 1974b; 1978).

Public School Experiences

The second author has worked in the public schools in Southern California for the past 20 years. Following are some clinical observations and experiences of treating preschool stuttering children in this environment. The number of all preschoolers with speech and language problems being treated in the public schools has gradually increased over the past years, probably due to the 1975 Public Law (PL) 94-142, Individuals with Disabilities Education Act, and subsequent laws extending the age of service downward. However, there has not been a corresponding proportional increase in the number of preschool children who stutter. Only an estimated 20 children have been seen by the second author in the past 20-year period of preschool service. (This number is an estimate because the second author changed schools several times and the children's records, by law, remained behind.)

It is estimated, in retrospect, that these stuttering children fell into two categories: (a) those with concurrent severe articulation and/or language problems (estimated 30%) and (b) those with stuttering problems only (estimated 70%). (This contrasts with the finding by Ryan, 1992, that none of the 20 stuttering preschool children in that study had a clinical language problem, although a few had articulation problems.)

All preschool children who stuttered were treated first with parent counseling, defined as giving the parents information about stuttering (e.g., 70% outgrow the problem) and simple suggestions for the parents to carry out at home. Although counseling is not considered an official part of the MFP per se, we have always given information to clients about stuttering in addition to treating them with the MFP. The second author then administered the Fluency Interview and speech and language tests periodically over time, followed by speech or language training, if indicated. Finally, if the stuttering problem did not disappear, the child was treated with the MFP: GILCU establishment, then transfer, and maintenance as described above (see Table 9-1).

Because it is often necessary in the U.S.A. public education system for parents to transport preschool children to the school where treatment is offered, they, and younger siblings, were often part of any speech evaluation. This permitted the second author to observe their interactions, an important part of any evaluation of a preschool child. Often parents of preschool children who stuttered, especially those with only a stuttering speech problem, were anxious about the problem. The child's preschool teacher or the grandparents frequently put pressure on the parents to "do something." For these parents, the counseling (usually with the mother, but more and more commonly these days, with fathers, too) always included telling the parents that 70% of children who stutter will outgrow the problem; then one or more of the following instructions, depending on what was observed during the evaluation, was given to the parents:

- Request and insure that the siblings who are talking for, or making it difficult for the client to get a chance to talk, permit the child to talk.
- Change their (parents') own speech (e.g., slow down, less talking, less complex talking).
- Avoid giving the child directions on how to talk fluently (e.g., "take a deep breath, think before you speak").
- Reduce the level of verbal activity and/or expectations (e.g., "Take it down one notch"). Ask fewer questions and accept less than perfect grammar and pronunciation.
- Reinforce (reward) fluent utterances with statements such as "I like how you told that story."
- Manage the environment to assure that the child does not feel rushed when talking.

A tacit effect of this counseling was that the second author was in contact with the parent and available for help from there on and would do more if the problems did not improve. The second author believes that this is a powerful therapeutic influence (i.e., "There is a doctor in the house").

EVALUATION OF THE PROGRAM

We have presented data, through publication and presentation of papers, on the efficacy and efficiency of the MFP for 291 clients treated by 229 student and professional clinicians (Ryan, 1971, 1974, 1981, 1985c, 1998c; Ryan & Ryan, 1983, 1994, 1995; Ryan & Van Kirk, 1974a, 1974b). The clients ranged in age from 4 to 66 and lived in Germany, Great Britain, Hong Kong, and the United States. The effectiveness of the program was demonstrated by the reduction of stuttering from a mean of 8.9 SW/M to less than a mean 0.5 SW/M for these clients, well within the range of normal fluency (Craven & Ryan, 1985). Follow-up of 11 clients conducted almost 5 years post-treatment indicated that most continued to speak fluently (Ryan, 1981).

The efficiency data of the MFP are that establishment usually took 8 hours of treatment, transfer 10 hours, and maintenance 2 hours, for a total of 20 hours of treatment (Rustin, Ryan, & Ryan, 1987; Ryan, 1971, 1998c; Ryan & Ryan, 1983, 1994, 1995; Ryan & Van Kirk, 1974a, 1974b). The program book (Ryan, 1985c; Ryan & Van Kirk, 1978) along with a training workshop provided clear descriptions of the procedures which resulted in replication of these results on three continents (Ryan, 1985c; Ryan & Ryan, 1994). The published data on the program also permitted the MFP to meet 10 of the 12 criteria for evaluation of treatment programs proposed by Bloodstein (1995, pp. 439-445) (Ryan, 1998c; Ryan & Ryan, 1994, 1998).

Before we evaluate the MFP for preschool children who stutter, we wish to restate that the desired outcome of this procedure for people who stutter is normally fluent speech, an attainable goal with preschool children who stutter because they do not have long histories of stuttering nor, based on our experiences and in our opinion, extensive outer (audience) or inner (self) negative reactions to it. However, even with these reasonable, high expectations of the efficacy of the treatment for preschoolers, evaluation of any treatment program for preschool children should still contain control for the possible occurrence of spontaneous recovery (Bloodstein, 1995; Curlee & Yairi, 1997; Ryan, 1984a, 1985a, 1990, 1993, 1998b; Ryan & Marsh, 1989; Yairi & Ambrose, 1992; Yairi, Ambrose, Paden, & Throneburg, 1996). One should obtain extensive pretreatment base rate data of stuttering to determine the direction and stability of the stuttering behavior (detect spontaneous recovery) before starting treatment, one of the many criteria for obtaining efficacy data on treatment programs for young children, according to Ingham and Riley (1998). Identification of children who will spontaneously recover is important so that they will not (a) be offered unnecessary treatment, nor (b) provide inflated positive, but false, efficacy data about treatment procedures employed with them. Repeated objective measurement of the preschool child's stuttering over time can often accurately predict its future course and aid in the selection of preschool children who need treatment (Ryan, 1984a, 1998b).

The provision of counseling before starting direct clinical treatment by the second author allowed for the occurrence, and hence detection, of possible spontaneous recovery. The second author observed that the most common result of continual counseling over several months was that all the children improved, many achieved normal fluency, but some persisted in stuttering at a noticeable level, and some even got worse after having improved.

In all six cases of children with multiple speech and language problems including stuttering, the result of treating the articulation and/or language, together with parent counseling, was the complete elimination of stuttering. The sample was admittedly small and the improvement in stuttering could have been attributed to spontaneous recovery. Parent counseling alone resolved the problem in five cases of children with stuttering problems only.

The remaining nine preschool stuttering children who persisted in stuttering and were on the MFP all achieved normal fluency as measured by repeated Fluency Interviews, observations in other settings, and reports by parents and/or preschool teachers. Follow-up suggested that the children had maintained their fluency over time. The results were often better than those achieved with older populations reported previously in the literature by us.

The experience of the first author with the Monterey Fluency Program with preschool children has been somewhat different due to his extensive longitudinal study (Ryan, 1984a, 1990, 1992, 1998a, 1998b; Ryan & Marsh, 1989), one of the goals of which was to find procedures to predict the spontaneous recovery of stuttering. To determine who would outgrow stuttering and who would not, none of the children received treatment immediately. When repeated measures over a year showed that 31% of the children did not outgrow stuttering (Ryan, 1998b), these children were offered treatment. Three were put on the MFP: GILCU establishment, transfer, and maintenance (see Table 9-1) administered by graduate students who achieved results similar to those described by us in the literature, except that the length of treatment was extended because of the severity of the stuttering and other factors (e.g., the program was over-written for preschoolers). Another 13 children were treated with experimental therapy programs, some similar to GILCU and some involving paused or slowed speech (Jones & Ryan, 1998; Wood & Ryan, in press). These results will be reported elsewhere (e.g., Ryan, 1998a).

Future Clinical Research

We obviously need more clinical research to clarify the role of speech and language problems in the evaluation and treatment of stuttering in preschool children. Although we are satisfied with our procedures for children as represented by our clinical trial data in the literature (e.g., Ryan & Ryan, 1995) and above, we do wonder about the relative merits of the various programs and procedures presented in this book and elsewhere. We are especially interested in procedures that are similar to ours in theory, rationale, and design (i.e., testable), for example, those reported in Chapter 5. Onslow, O'Brian, and Harrison (1997) reported great improvement in stuttering to less than 1% SS in an average 10.5 hours of clinician time employing parents with minimal clinician involvement. This is an efficacious, especially efficient, procedure compared to our finding of a mean of 20 hours of treatment.

We will never know the efficacy of procedures that are ill-described, cannot be replicated, and/or have no objective efficacy data (Ingham & Riley, 1998), but it is our understanding of efficacy that after one has established the efficacy of a particular procedure, as we (e.g., Ryan & Ryan, 1995) or Onslow et al. (1997) have done, a next step is to compare this procedure with other verified procedures so that the more efficacious and/or efficient procedures may be identified (Ryan, 1974; Ryan & Ryan, 1983, 1994, 1995). Is the Lidcombe Program better than the MFP? Clinical trials research could answer this question. Or there may also be some future, as yet undiscovered or developed procedure, perhaps involving speaking rate (Wood & Ryan, in press), or other procedures described in this book, which may be the best treatment of stuttering in preschool children. Finally, we need to effectively and efficiently disseminate (Ryan, 1985c) the best procedures to our colleagues so that we as a profession may offer a uniform, efficacious procedure to the clearly treatable pre-school population of people who stutter.

SUMMARY

- When working with preschool children who stutter it is important to attempt to sort out the estimated 30% who will not outgrow the problem and offer them treatment
- The role of coexisting severe articulation and language problems and their consequent treatment in preschool children who stutter needs further investigation and clarification in the treatment of stuttering.
- The MFP, with appropriate revisions, may be used effectively and efficiently with preschool children who stutter in a wide variety of settings, including the public schools.
- It is necessary to describe treatment clearly and to collect objective, reliable, and valid data to establish the efficacy and efficiency of any procedure used with preschool children who stutter, at the least a measure of stuttering itself before and after treatment, and the hours of treatment.
- Preliminary results have been positive with a high percentage of complete elimination of stuttering in preschool children who clearly did not outgrow the problem, suggesting that it is appropriate and efficacious to treat preschool stuttering children directly.
- Further clinical trial research is needed to improve the present procedures and to discover the most efficacious procedures for preschool children who stutter.

REFERENCES

Bloodstein, O. (1995). *A handbook on stuttering* (5th ed.). San Diego, CA: Singular Publishing Group.

Craig, A., Hancock, K., Chang, E., McCready, C., Shepley, A., McCaul, A., Costello, D., Harding, S., Kehren, R., Masel, C., & Reily, K. (1996). A controlled clinical trial for stuttering in persons aged 9–14. *Journal of Speech and Hearing Research, 39,* 808–826.

Craven, D., & Ryan, B. (1985, November). *Disfluent behavior of normal speakers: Three modes of reading, monologue, and conversation.* Paper presented at the annual American Speech-Language-Hearing Convention, Washington, DC.

Curlee, R., & Yairi, E. (1997). Early intervention with early childhood stuttering: A critical examination of the data. *American Journal of Speech-Language Pathology, 6,* 8–18.

Fowler, S., & Ingham, R. (1986). Stuttering treatment rating recorder (STRR) (Version 2.0) [Computer program]. Santa Barbara: University of California at Santa Barbara.

Ingham, J., & Riley, G. (1998). Guidelines for documentation of treatment efficacy for young children who stutter. *Journal of Speech, Language and Hearing Research, 41*, 753-770.

Ingham, R. (1984). *Stuttering and behavior therapy: Current status and experimental foundations.* San Diego, CA: College-Hill Press.

Johnson, W. (1961). Measurements of oral reading and speaking rate and disfluency of adult male and female stutterers and nonstutterers. *Journal of Speech and Hearing Disorders, 7*(Suppl.), 1–20.

Jones, P., & Ryan, B. (1998). *Experimental analysis of the relationship between speaking and stuttering rate during mother-child conversation.* Manuscript submitted for publication.

Onslow, M., Adams, R., & Ingham, R. (1992). Reliability of speech naturalness ratings of stuttered speech during treatment. *Journal of Speech and Hearing Research, 35*, 994–1001.

Onslow, M., O'Brian, S., & Harrison, E. (1997). The Lidcombe Program of early stuttering intervention: Methods and issues. *European Journal of Disorders of Communication, 32*, 231–250.

Pipe, P. (1966). *Practical programming.* New York: Holt, Rinehart, and Winston.

Rustin, L., Ryan, B., & Ryan, B. (1987). Use of the Monterey programmed stuttering treatment in Great Britain. *British Journal of Disorders of Communication, 22*, 151–162.

Ryan, B. (1971). Operant procedures applied to stuttering treatment for children. *Journal of Speech and Hearing Disorders, 36*, 264–280.

Ryan, B. (1974). *Programmed stuttering treatment for children and adults.* Springfield, IL: Charles C. Thomas.

Ryan, B. (1981). Maintenance programs in progress—II. In E. Boberg (Ed.), *Maintenance of fluency* (pp. 113–146). New York: Elsevier.

Ryan, B. (1984a, November). *A comparison/longitudinal study of the development of stuttering.* Paper presented at the Annual Convention of the American Speech-Language-Hearing Association, San Francisco, CA.

Ryan, B. (1984b). Treatment of stuttering in school children. In W. Perkins (Ed.), *Current treatment of communication disorders: Stuttering disorders* (pp. 95–106). New York: Thieme-Stratton.

Ryan, B. (1985a, November). *A comparison/longitudinal study of the development of stuttering: Report 2.* Paper presented at the Annual Convention of the American Speech-Language-Hearing Association, Washington, DC.

Ryan, B. (1985b). Operant procedures applied to stuttering treatment for children. In G. Shames & H. Rubin (Eds.), *Stuttering then and now* (pp. 417–443). Columbus, OH: Charles E. Merrill.

Ryan, B. (1985c). Training the professional. *Seminars in Speech and Language, 6*, 145–168.

Ryan, B. (1990). *A comparison/longitudinal study of the development of stuttering: Report 4*. Paper presented at the Annual Convention of the American Speech-Language-Hearing Association, Seattle, WA. (Abstract published in *Asha, 32,* 144)

Ryan, B. (1992). Articulation, language, rate, and fluency characteristics of 20 stuttering and nonstuttering preschool children. *Journal of Speech and Hearing Research, 35,* 333–342.

Ryan, B. (1993, November). *A comparison/longitudinal study of the development of stuttering: Report 5*. Paper presented at the Annual Convention of the American Speech-Language-Hearing Association, Anaheim, CA.

Ryan, B. (1998a). Efficacy research to develop treatment programs for preschool children who stutter. In A. Cordes & R. Ingham (Eds.), *Toward efficacy for stuttering treatment: A search for empirical bases* (pp. 163–190). San Diego, CA: Singular Publishing Group.

Ryan, B. (1998b). *A longitudinal study of articulation, language, rate, and fluency of 22 preschool children who stuttered*. Unpublished manuscript.

Ryan, B. (1998c). *Speaking rate, conversational speech acts, and linguistic complexity of 20 preschool stuttering and nonstuttering children and their mothers*. Manuscript submitted for publication.

Ryan, B., & Marsh, C. (1989, November). *A comparison/longitudinal study of the development of stuttering: Report 3*. Paper presented at the Annual Convention of the American Speech-Language-Hearing Association, New Orleans, LA.

Ryan, B., & Ryan, B. (1983). Programmed treatment for children: Comparison of four programs. *Journal of Fluency Disorders, 8,* 291–321.

Ryan, B., & Ryan, B. (1994). *Monterey fluency program: A retrospective*. Paper presented at the First World Congress of Fluency Disorders, Munich, Germany. (Abstract published in *Journal of Fluency Disorders, 19,* 206)

Ryan, B., & Ryan, B. (1995). Programmed stuttering treatment for children: Comparison of two establishment programs, through transfer, maintenance, and follow-up. *Journal of Speech and Hearing Research, 38,* 61–75.

Ryan, B., & Ryan, B. (1998). *The Monterey fluency program: A study in efficacy*. Unpublished manuscript.

Ryan, B., & Van Kirk, B. (1971). *Programmed conditioning for fluency*. Monterey, CA: Behavioral Sciences Institute.

Ryan, B., & Van Kirk, B. (1973). *Counting disfluencies, stuttered words, and total words* [A tape recorded training program]. Monterey, CA: Monterey Learning Systems.

Ryan, B., & Van Kirk, B. (1974a). *Programmed stuttering treatment for children* (Final report, Office of Education Project 0-72-4422). Washington, DC: U.S. Department of Health, Education and Welfare.

Ryan, B., & Van Kirk, B. (1974b). The establishment, transfer, and maintenance of fluent speech in 50 stutterers using delayed auditory feedback and operant procedures. *Journal of Speech and Hearing Research, 39,* 3–10.

Ryan, B., & Van Kirk, B. (1978). *Monterey Fluency Program.* Monterey, CA: Monterey Learning Systems.

Silverman, F. (1995). Can disfluencies be categorized reliably using Wendell Johnson's scheme? *Journal of Speech and Hearing Research, 38,* 586.

Takata, S. (1989). *Mothers' ability to scale the stuttering severity of their preschool children.* Unpublished master's thesis. California State University, Long Beach, CA.

Wood, M., & Ryan, B. (in press). Experimental analysis of speaking and stuttering rate in a child who stutters. *Journal of Developmental and Physical Disabilities.*

Yairi, E., & Ambrose, N. (1992). A longitudinal study of stuttering in children: A preliminary report. *Journal of Speech and Hearing Research, 35,* 755–760.

Yairi, E., Ambrose, N., Paden, E., & Throneburg, R. (1996). Predictive factors of persistence and recovery: Pathways of childhood stuttering. *Journal of Communication Disorders, 29,* 51–77.

10

Treatment of Early Stuttering: Some Reflections

JOSEPH S. ATTANASIO

INTRODUCTION

The focus of this chapter is summation. That is, the task is to sum up the text and offer concluding comments. A secondary task is to draw conclusions about the state of the art in early intervention in stuttering. Such tasks are not to be undertaken lightly. First, there is the danger of misrepresenting the words and intentions of the authors who have contributed chapters, while at the same time giving them no opportunity to respond (see Curlee & Perkins, 1984, preface). Second, there is the danger of bias and partiality in the comments that follow. It is not the purpose of this chapter, however, to critique any of the approaches in order to recommend one or more of them; all are recommended for consideration. Finally, any attempt to draw conclusions about the state of the art early intervention risks the omission of points of view that are not expressed in the preceding chapters. Despite the dangers and risks, it is appropriate to respond to and comment on the material presented in the text. Perhaps the justification for doing so is to express what readers of the text might have said if given a chance, or to open a dialogue by proxy. Readers of the text, therefore, are invited to think about the ideas that have been presented in the text, and that are offered in the comments that follow, and to formulate their own reactions and opinions. More to the point, however, is the hope that clinicians will gain increased confidence and skill in assisting young children who stutter as a result of studying what the authors offer.

This chapter proceeds in its tasks by abstracting and focusing on several themes that run through the text: (1) the role of theory in the treatment programs, (2) perspectives on treatment common to the programs, and (3) thorny issues, or questions that are not fully resolved.

EARLY INTERVENTION IN STUTTERING

The Role of Theory

A good starting point for summing up and for opening a dialogue is to state what the text is about as well as what it is not about. To do so helps to establish a context for the text within the existing literature on the treatment of early stuttering. It is clear from the text's title that its purpose is to describe approaches to intervention strategies for early stuttering. Each of its chapters contains practical suggestions that have direct clinical application. It is likewise clear from the content of each of the chapters that we are not presented with scientific theories of the distal or, in some cases, not even the proximal causes of stuttering. Scientific theories generate testable hypotheses and make predictions that can be verified by observation. Some of the chapter authors, however, might argue that they have explicated theories of cause or that their treatment programs are theoretically based. Let us see.

Pindzola's Stuttering Intervention Program (Chapter 6) is based on her clinical experiences, insights, and a collection of research studies that, while not challenged here, do not represent a unified theory strictly defined. The Monterey Fluency Program (Chapter 9), the Lidcombe Program (Chapter 5), and, in part, the Stuttering Intervention Program (Chapter 6) are based on the related concepts of operant conditioning, programmed instruction, and behavior modification. By definition, operant methodologies are typically atheoretical (Onslow, 1996).

Conture and Melnick's Parent-Child Group Approach (Chapter 2) and Gottwald and Starkweather's Multiprocess Approach (Chapter 3) use principles and notions born of their clinical experiences and their interpretations of the research literature that, although intuitively appealing as explanations of stuttering, remain assumptions that require the development of testable hypotheses and experimental evidence. Indeed, Stark-weather and Gottwald (1990) have indicated that the Demands and Capacities model is actually not a scientific model. Riley and Riley's Speech Motor Training (7) and, to some extent, the Fluency Rules Program by Runyan and Runyan (Chapter 8) are physiologically based. For example, Riley and Riley's program aims to improve speech motor production as a way to reduce stuttering frequency and severity and is derived from the principles of oral motor training; certain aspects of the Fluency Rules Program focus on the physiologic behaviors of breathing and laryngeal activity. The Fluency Rules Program, however, was generated from therapy principles and validated from observations of its clinical effectiveness without actual attempts to theorize on the nature or cause of stuttering. Perhaps Riley and Riley's program in speech motor training provides the closest attempt to base intervention on theory and, in turn, to test the predictions that the theory makes. That is, Riley and Riley state that their program is based on the principles of Stetson's motor phonetics, and they present research findings in stuttering that point to problems in speech motor production and control. In the end, a distinction has to be made between basing clinical intervention on research and basing it on theory; not all research is theoretically driven.

Having dispatched any claim that the intervention programs presented in the text are truly based on scientific theory, it is only fair to state that the absence of theoretical underpinnings does not cast doubt on the clinical effectiveness of the intervention programs. Nor do the preceding comments on theory deny the successes that the authors report for their programs. Given the reported effectiveness of the programs described in the text, clinicians can no longer suggest to themselves or to others that there is little to do for treating early stuttering or, worse yet, that nothing should be done. Theory may not be necessary for effective therapy (Perkins, 1986), and clinicians have daily success with their clients while working outside the context of theory. The text is a testament to the fact that clinical intervention for early stuttering may proceed while the important work of finding the cause or causes of stuttering continues.

It would be misleading, however, to imply that there is complete consensus on the need to provide direct treatment to all children with early stuttering without considering the possibility of unaided remission. Unaided remission is a thorny issue and is addressed later in this chapter.

Common Ground

What, then, do these programs offer? Is there common ground, despite the obvious differences among the programs? Both questions are answered in the sections that follow.

The Need for Early Intervention

It is clear from reading the text that early intervention for stuttering is possible, necessary, and effective. While the debate on spontaneous or unaided remission of stuttering and on the actual percentage of remission to be expected continues (see Curlee & Yairi, 1997), the programs in the text and the research on which they are based indicate that intervention for early stuttering is appropriate for a great number of children.

Direct Intervention

Furthermore, direct intervention is appropriate for many children. That is, in one way or another, the programs described in the text do not refrain from calling children's attention to their speech, their fluency, and their stuttering. Indeed, a number of years ago, Wingate (1959) found that stuttering decreased when it was called to the attention of the person who stuttered. Siegel (1970) severely damaged the position that punishing stuttering would make it worse. A striking example that weakens the notion that punishment worsens stuttering and at the same time suggests that punishment may in fact reduce stuttering is what has come to be called "the puppet study" (Martin, Kuhl, & Haroldson 1972). Martin et al. created a situation in which two preschool-age children separately conversed with a puppet that was operated by the experimenter in another room. Time-out from talking was administered contingent on stuttering: the puppet stopped conversing with the children and the area around the puppet was darkened, causing it to "disappear." Both children evidenced an immediate reduction in stuttering when compared to baseline conditions, and the reductions generalized to conversational sessions with an adult in the laboratory. Time-out may be seen as a form of punishment, in that it is known to reduce stuttering. Within the context of operant methodology, punishment is a stimulus that reduces or eliminates the future occurrence of the behavior it follows or is contingent on. Although there was some indication from Martin et al. that the increased fluency was maintained after 1 year, caution is needed in interpreting the results because it is not clear that time-out was the actual agent that caused the stuttering to lessen and because the results have not been replicated (Onslow, 1996).

Clinicians' acceptance of findings such as those of Wingate (1959), Siegel (1970), and Martin et al. (1972) has been slow in coming, as has been the development of intervention programs for early stuttering that directly call the child's attention to the processes of speech and to the attributes of fluency and stuttering. However, a hopeful sign has been documented in a survey by Cooper and Cooper (1996). A comparison of the results of a survey done between 1983 and 1991 with those of a survey taken between 1973 and 1983 indicated an increase in the number of clinicians (though by far not the majority) who believed that children should be made aware of their stuttering as part of treatment, regardless of the children's ages (Cooper & Cooper, 1996). The Lidcombe Program (Chapter 5) and the Stuttering Intervention Program (Chapter 6) are the approaches presented in the text that most obviously use the principles of calling attention to fluency by rewarding it and, conversely, calling attention to stuttering by correcting it when it occurs. Riley and Riley's Speech Motor Training (Chapter 7), however, does focus exclusively on speech by guiding the child in the acquisition of detailed and specific control of speech motor production.

Response-Contingent Stimulation

Five of the programs use response-contingent stimulation (RCS) to reduce or eliminate stuttering. The use of RCS is obvious in the Stuttering Intervention Program, the Monterey Fluency Program, and the Lidcombe Program. To a lesser extent, RCS is used in the Speech Motor Training program and in the Fluency Rules Program. In the present context, RCS is a procedure that provides an environmental consequence (stimulus) contingent on the occurrence of a speech act (response). The consequence or stimulus is typically provided by a parent or clinician, taking the form of either positive reinforcement of fluent speech or correction (punishment) of stuttered speech. The child may be praised for fluent speech or corrected for stuttered speech by being asked to stop and repeat the utterance without the stuttering. In the Lidcombe Program, for example, the child may be told, "that was good talking, there were no 'bumps'" when speech was fluent and "I heard 'bumps,' say that again without the 'bumps'" when speech was stuttered. In addition, time-out from talking (TO), a form of RCS, can be seen in the Stuttering Intervention Program and the Monterey Fluency Program. It is used to a lesser extent in the Stuttering Prevention and Early Intervention programs.

The Environment

Several of the programs in the text incorporate what has come to be called "the environmental hypothesis" (Cox, Seider, & Kidd, 1984) and attempt to alter the child's environment as one way to increase fluency and decrease stuttering. Other programs do not. All of the programs, however, make it clear that, for a number of children (perhaps most, but the data are not in as yet), environmental manipulation is not sufficient to eliminate stuttering or reduce its occurrence and that some form of direct intervention on the child's speech must take place. Said another way, environmental change may be necessary, at least in some of the programs, but is not seen as sufficient in any of the programs.

The role of the environment in the etiology and maintenance of stuttering remains a thorny issue and is considered further later in this chapter. It may be instructive, however, to make a distinction between two forms of environmental manipulation, indirect and direct. Gottwald and Starkweather's program provides an excellent example of indirect environmental manipulation in which attempts are made to increase or enhance children's capacities for fluency and to decrease the demands for fluency that are placed on them. Factors that are manipulated are embedded within interacting environmental systems (e.g., the family, the school, and the neighborhood) and in the children themselves. The Lidcombe Program provides an excellent example of direct environmental manipulation. The Lidcombe Program is based on operant methodology directed primarily at the child's speech, but it does in fact manipulate the environment. When a parent provides reinforcement for fluent speech and correction for stuttered speech, the child's environment has been manipulated or changed in some way. Counseling for parents is directed primarily at how best to arrange the environment for the effective administration of response-contingent stimulation. The distinctions between indirect and direct environmental manipulation are analogous to the distinctions between indirect and direct treatment made by Ingham and Cordes (1998). According to Ingham and Cordes, indirect treatment focuses on environmental or parental behaviors, whereas direct treatment focuses on the child's speech behaviors.

Multidimensional Intervention

All of the programs share the notion that intervention is multidimensional rather than unidimensional. That is, intervention makes use of multiple procedures, concepts, or hierarchies. While at first blush the use of multiple procedures and concepts may be viewed as a strength, on closer examination, a liability eventually is discernible. Researchers call that liability multiple treatment interference (Schiavetti & Metz, 1997) when discussing threats to the external validity of treatment research studies. With reference to the clinical efficacy of treatment programs, multiple treatment interference refers to the difficulty of determining the extent to which the multiple procedures of a given program interact with each other to produce reduced stuttering or increased fluency. It becomes quite difficult to know the separate effects of each procedure in a multiple procedures approach and whether or not each and every procedure is actually necessary for the reduction of stuttering or the increase of fluency. A similar problem may be seen in programs that use a hierarchical approach. For these programs, the question is whether or not the hierarchy is necessary for all children in order for the intervention to be successful.

Related to the notion of multidimensional intervention is the issue of stuttering etiology as multifactorial or interactional. Multifactorial or interactionist modeling of stuttering's etiology is another of those thorny issues which is discussed later in this chapter.

Duration of Treatment

It is important to note that none of the programs imply that intervention for early stuttering is simply a matter of applying a "quick fix." Quite the contrary. All of the programs, whether based on nonbehavioral or behavioral methodologies, make it clear that intervention is a long-term process that may last a year or more.

Data Collection

It is heartening to see that so many of the programs require the collection of objective and reliable clinical data, often in the form of number of syllables stuttered per unit of time or percent stuttering per unit of time or per speech unit, as a measure of client progress or program effectiveness. If reduced stuttering or increased fluency are goals of treatment, as they are for many of the programs described in the text, then outcomes measures should be in a form that verifies reduced stuttering or increased fluency through the collection of objective and reliable data both within and beyond the clinical setting. All too often in the past, measurement for outcomes purposes has been vague and ill-defined. Judgments of treatment outcomes in other disorder areas have become more specific and so must those for stuttering. In the case of articulation or phonology disorders, for example, it would be unusual for clinicians not to count the number of correct articulations of target sounds or to chart increases in the percentage of correct productions. With voice disorders, to give a second example, instrumentation is available to assess such factors as changes in the size of a vocal lesion or the adequacy of subglottal air pressure; instrumentation is used in conjunction with perceptual judgments. Although outcomes measurement in other disorder areas is not without problems, attempts to refine and improve those measures are ongoing. Therein, however, lies another thorny issue for treatment outcomes in stuttering. That is, criteria for success are somewhat uneven across programs. This issue is addressed next.

Thorny Issues

Unaided Remission

Curlee and Yairi (1997) expressed the opinion that the question of the need to treat every child who stutters as soon as possible after onset remains unanswered, specifically for children who are between 2 and 5 years of age and who have been stuttering between 1 and 2 years. An exception would be made for children who show negative reactions to their stuttering or whose parents want the children treated. Furthermore, Curlee and Yairi maintain that delaying treatment for these children does not limit the effectiveness of intervention for children for whom it becomes necessary and that monitoring children during the first 2 years of stuttering onset prior to intervention allows for unaided remission to take place, which they suggest will occur for most of the children. Curlee and Yairi reached their conclusions despite widespread agreement in the literature they reviewed that early intervention for young children who stutter, when compared to treatment outcomes for older children and adults, results in more frequent and longer lasting generalization of fluent speech, more cases of permanent remission, and requires fewer hours of treatment. Curlee and Yairi cited problems of research design and methodology in that literature.

Yet, data presented by Ingham and Cordes (1998) make a strong case for not delaying treatment. Ingham and Cordes found that 81.8% of preschool children treated for stuttering had a satisfactory outcome based on criteria established by the authors, but only 54.2% of school-age children treated for stuttering did so. These differences are consistent with data Ingham and Cordes (1998) presented in another comparison. Eighty-five percent of children who received treatment within 15 months of onset reached criteria, but criteria were reached by only 59.4% of children for whom treatment was delayed beyond 15 months postonset. Similar findings, Ingham and Cordes suggested, can be found in other reports of early versus delayed treatment. Taken together, these reports may be seen as replication of the finding that the chance for successful treatment outcome is greater for younger children. They support the view that early treatment is desirable.

The foregoing discussion on unaided remission has several implications for the programs in this text and for clinicians who are faced with intervention decisions for young children who stutter. First, the very concept of unaided remission must be questioned. To suggest that remission is unaided is to suggest that there is sufficient evidence to support the notion that parents or other individuals in the child's environment do nothing or say nothing to modify the child's speech while monitoring is taking place. Such evidence is lacking and there is reason to believe that parents of children who reportedly experience unaided remission make use of treatment techniques of their own (Martin & Lindamood, 1986). Second, Curlee and Yairi's reasoning may be based on research that has not employed all of the methodology available to help distinguish treatment effects from the effects of unaided remission (see Ingham & Cordes, 1998). Third, there is evidence that early intervention is not harmful to children and that, consequently, it may be better to intervene and risk false positive identification and treatment than to risk false negative identification and by so doing delay treatment unnecessarily (Onslow, 1992). Finally, the issue of remission is not ignored by the authors in this book. For example, a 3-month testing or monitoring period before initiating treatment is built into the Monterey Fluency Program (Chapter 9). Conture and Melnick (Chapter 2) attempt to be reasonably certain that stuttering will not remit before they begin to treat the young child, while

Gottwald and Starkweather (Chapter 3) acknowledge the issue of remission and point to the use of known risk factors in the decision to begin treatment, but also state that there is strong support to treat any preschool child who is stuttering.

Ingham and Cordes (1998) echo the view that, whenever treatment for early stuttering is delayed for given children, the waiting period is to be used for data collection by parents and clinicians in a variety of situations so that a careful and data-based analysis can be made of increases or decreases in stuttering. Ingham and Cordes (1998) suggest that monitoring the child's speech in that way is quite different from simply waiting to see if spontaneous remission will occur. At the heart of the views of Ingham and Cordes, however, is their belief that neither our professional ethics nor our accumulated data on early stuttering support the tactic of withholding treatment for early stuttering.

The issue of remission is not limited to stuttering. We struggle with it, for example, when we are faced with the decision to treat young children with articulation or language disorders. Speech-language pathologists have had normative data on speech sound acquisition available to them for quite some time. However, knowing that most children acquire a given speech sound by a given age does not translate into knowing if an individual child will acquire that sound at the age indicated in the normative data. By definition, norms are developed from the study of population samples and are actuarial in nature; they are in the form of probability statements based on the behaviors of groups. A mistake is made if we suggest that, because the normative data indicate that 90% of children acquire a given skill (e.g., speech sound acquisition) at a given age, an individual child has a 90% chance of acquiring that skill at that age. Bernstein-Ratner (1997) makes a similar point when discussing the remission of early stuttering. It remains an inescapable fact of professional life that speech-language pathologists need to supplement the normative data available to them with other sources of information when making treatment decisions.

The Environmental Hypothesis

The role of the environment in the etiology or maintenance of stuttering and, by extension, the use of environmental change in intervention programs, continues to be problematic. Typically, when the environment is seen as a factor in stuttering, attention is focused on the child's communicative environment (Kloth, Janssen, Kraaimaat, & Brutten, 1995). Implicated are the parents' speech patterns, the pace of communication, and the competition for speaking. Several of the programs in this text pay some attention to one or all of those aspects of the child's environment. It is intuitively appealing to believe that the speech environment that surrounds the child plays some part in the etiology or maintenance of stuttering. The same intuition applies to other childhood disorders of communication such as language delay and articulation. To think otherwise borders on heresy.

Cox et al. (1984), however, in their study of environmental factors and stuttering, found little evidence to support the environmental hypothesis. Specifically, they concluded that particular parental attitudes, high anxiety levels in families of individuals who stutter, and poor family attitudes toward speech were not causally linked to stuttering or its development. Interestingly, Cox et al. used what they termed "high density stuttering families," defined as families in which there were "at least five individuals who reported or exhibited stuttering for at least 6 consecutive months" (Cox et al., 1984).

In their review of the literature, Nippold and Rudzinski (1995) reached two conclusions that directly affect intervention programs that encourage changes in parental speech behaviors: (a) parents of children who stutter do not differ in the way they talk with their children when compared to parents of children who do not stutter and (b) parental speech behaviors do not contribute to stuttering in children. Kloth et al. (1995) conducted a prospective study which led them to suggest that the communicative behaviors of mothers of children who were at risk for developing stuttering because of family history but who were normally fluent at the start of the study do not contribute to the development of stuttering. Mothers' communicative style and speaking rate did not causally relate to the development of stuttering. However, the complexity of mothers' language, as measured by mean length of utterance (MLU), did distinguish children who went on to stutter and those who did not. Curiously, the mothers of children who developed stuttering used language that was less complex at the beginning of the study than did the mothers of children who did not develop stuttering. This last finding is counterintuitive when one considers prevailing wisdom.

In the end, intervention programs that give a role to environmental manipulation or change in the remediation of stuttering must address more completely the issues raised in the research reviewed above on environmental factors. In the meantime, clinicians must be aware that there is not sufficient evidence to believe that parental speech behaviors contribute to stuttering or that those speech behaviors must be modified in order for children to gain increased fluency (Nippold & Rudzinski, 1995).

Intervention programs based on operant methodology are no less susceptible to the problematic nature of the relationship of the environment to stuttering. In the chapter by Lincoln and Harrison (Chapter 5), the view is taken that, although environmental events do not cause stuttering, environmental consequences can control stuttering. That is, stuttering has operant-like properties and may be reduced or eliminated through the administration of response-contingent stimulation. That very premise requires further explanation. How can it be that while stuttering is not caused by environmental influences it can be controlled by environmental contingencies once it has started? A full answer is needed.

A considerable part of this chapter has been devoted to the issue of the role of the communicative environment in stuttering because of the prominent place it has held in the thinking on stuttering and its origins and maintenance. The firm hold that the environmental hypothesis has had on our thinking has been weakened, but not yet put aside, if indeed it ever will or should be.

Multifactorial or Interactionist Models

Multifactorial or interactionist models posit that, for any given child, many factors contribute to stuttering and that these factors (innate and environmental) interact with one another to cause stuttering. Thus, multifactorial is seen as multicausal (Packman, Onslow, & Attanasio, 1997). Intervention programs (e.g., Gottwald & Starkweather, Chapter 3) based on such models operate on, or address, the various factors and their interactions in the attempt to decrease stuttering and increase fluency. Multifactorial models of stuttering reflect the notion that stuttering is a complex disorder. Accepting the observation that developed stuttering is complex in its manifestations, however, does not make it axiomatic that the causes of stuttering are complex or that intervention must be. To do so may be to evoke what is known as reasoning by representativeness, or the representativeness heuristic. Applied to stuttering, the heuristic suggests that, if the observable phenomena of stuttering are complex, so too must be their causes. It is a case of reasoning back from effects to causes. There is obvious danger in doing so (Attanasio, Onslow, & Packman, 1998). Multifactorial models need experimentally testable hypotheses and demonstrations of their explanatory power (Packman et al., 1997) to support the view that stuttering and its treatment must be multifactorial in nature. It is not being suggested here that the successes achieved through multifactorial intervention programs for early stuttering are not real. Rather, the suggestion is similar to the one made in reference to multiple treatment interference: We must know just what is and is not necessary for successful treatment so that our intervention efforts can be efficient and, especially in the case of early stuttering, timely. It may turn out, for example, that the time spent on modifying or manipulating factors that do not reduce or eliminate stuttering in young children (see the discussion above on parental speech) diverts attention from those factors that do. Precious time may be wasted.

Outcome Criteria

There are instances in the text where success is defined as stuttering that is within normal limits. Such a criterion raises the question of what is meant by the term stuttering. Is stuttering ever normal? Is stuttering the same as normal nonfluency? Of course, this is the issue of definition. Other programs in the text define success in the presence of residual stuttering; for some, less than 1% is acceptable, while for others less than 3% is acceptable. At least one program (Conture & Melnick, Chapter 2) does not aim for specific fluency criteria but rather for improved communication; speech that is completely free from stuttering is not the goal.

As this chapter is being written, the profession of speech-language pathology is making a concerted effort to find ways to measure the outcomes of treatment programs for a variety of communication disorders and to develop methods to determine the efficacy of treatment. That is no small undertaking. Because it is not the purpose here to review outcomes or efficacy models, the reader is encouraged to consult the available literature and texts.

The differences in the outcome criteria used in the programs described in this text point to at least three questions that should be considered in evaluating those programs: (a) are the criteria clearly stated and can they be used to assess the program's success in reaching the goals set for or by the person who stutters? (b) do the criteria match the point of view about the nature and treatment of stuttering taken by the program? And perhaps most importantly (c) are the criteria grounded in a well-defined rationale that speaks to the day-to-day communicative needs of the individual? It may well be that our clients ultimately define success, for they must be satisfied with themselves as communicators.

CONCLUDING COMMENTS

The variety of the intervention strategies for early stuttering offered in this book may at first overwhelm the reader because of the diversity of the viewpoints represented. Indeed, clinicians may be heard to complain that they find such diversity confusing and that they therefore despair of knowing what to do for their young clients who stutter. That very diversity, however, signifies that there is much that can be done to reduce or eliminate early stuttering or improve communication. The days of the "wait and watch" approach to early stuttering are over. Indeed, Nippold and Rudzinski (1995) have called such an approach "dangerous" and cautioned against intervention practices that focus solely on parent counseling and limited clinician/child contact. Given the variety of approaches from indirect to direct offered in this book, the "wait and watch" approach is no longer a reasonable option to take with many children. There are approaches here that will suit the most cautious of clinicians and others that will resonate for clinicians who adopt direct intervention strategies.

Rather than be overwhelmed, then, readers can be reassured that the clinical armamentarium contains a richness of approaches that can accommodate what they believe about stuttering and that can meet the needs of their clients. At the same time, careful reading of the text will disclose an organizing principle: there appears to be a finite number of things that need to be done to reduce stuttering. Rather than being a reflection of our limitations, that finiteness of treatment options is a reflection of the ongoing distillation of our attempts to develop effective intervention strategies for early stuttering. By no means, however, is the task finished. It is for clinicians to decide, after thoughtful reflection, which of the approaches described in the text are appropriate to their work and for their clients at this point in our professional journey.

REFERENCES

Attansio, J. S., Onslow, M., & Packman, A. (1998). Representativeness reasoning and the search for origins of stuttering: A return to basic observations. *Journal of Fluency Disorders, 23,* 265–274.
Bernstein-Ratner, N. (1997). Leaving Las Vegas: Clinical odds and individual outcomes. *American Journal of Speech-Language Pathology, 6,* 29–33.

Cooper, E. B., & Cooper, C. S. (1996). Clinician attitudes towards stuttering: Two decades of change. *Journal of Fluency Disorders, 21,* 119–135.

Cox, N. J., Seider, R. A., & Kidd, K. K. (1984). Some environmental factors and hypotheses for stuttering in families with several stutterers. *Journal of Speech and Hearing Research, 27,* 543–548.

Curlee, R. F., & Perkins, W. H. (Eds.). (1984). *Nature and treatment of stuttering: New directions.* San Diego: College-Hill Press.

Curlee, R. F., & Yairi, E. (1997). Early intervention with early childhood stuttering: A critical examination of the data. *American Journal of Speech-Language Pathology, 6,* 8–18.

Ingham, R. J., & Cordes, A. K. (1998). Treatment decisions for young children who stutter: Further concerns and complexities. *American Journal of Speech-Language Pathology, 7,* 10–19.

Kloth, S. A. M., Janssen, P., Kraaimaat, F. W., & Brutten, G. J. (1995). Communicative behavior of mothers of stuttering and nonstuttering high-risk children prior to the onset of stuttering. *Journal of Fluency Disorders, 20,* 365–377.

Martin, R. R., Kuhl, P., & Haroldson, S. (1972). An experimental treatment with two preschool stuttering children. *Journal of Speech and Hearing Research, 15,* 743–752.

Martin, R. R., & Lindamood, L. P. (1986). Stuttering and spontaneous recovery: Implications for the speech-language pathologist. *Language, Speech and Hearing Services in Schools, 17,* 207–218.

Nippold, M. A., & Rudzinski, M. (1995). Parents' speech and children's stuttering: A critique of the literature. *Journal of Speech and Hearing Research, 38,* 978–989.

Onslow, M. (1992). Identification of early stuttering: Issues and suggested strategies. *American Journal of Speech-Language Pathology, 1,* 21–27.

Onslow, M. (1996). *Behavioral management of stuttering.* San Diego, CA: Singular Publishing Group.

Packman, A., Onslow, M., & Attanasio, J. (1997). Multifactorial does not necessarily mean multicausal. Abstracts of the Second World Congress on Fluency Disorders [Special ed.] *Journal of Fluency Disorders, 22.*

Perkins, W. H. (1986). Functions and malfunctions of theories in therapies. *Asha, 28,* 31–33.

Schiavetti, N., & Metz, D. E. (1997). *Evaluating research in communicative disorders.* Boston: Allyn and Bacon.

Siegel, G. M. (1970). Punishment, stuttering, and disfluency. *Journal of Speech and Hearing Research, 4,* 677–714.

Starkweather, C. W., & Gottwald, S. R. (1990). The demands and capacities model: II. Clinical implications. *Journal of Fluency Disorders, 15,* 143–157.

Wingate, M. E. (1959). Calling attention to stuttering. *Journal of Speech and Hearing Research, 2,* 326–335.

Index

A

Abnormal disfluencies, 18

Abnormal syllable production, clinical skills required to recognize, 144–145

Accurate voicing, 148

Acoustic duration studies, 141–142

Analyzing child's speech, language, and fluency skills, 62–66

Assessment
  and evaluation of stuttering, 25–27
  of Lidcombe program, 105
  of multiprocess approach program
    analyzing child's speech, language, and fluency skills, 62–66
    collecting information prior to evaluation, 58–59
    collecting speech samples for analysis, 60
    interviewing family and preschool staff, 59–60
    measuring speech and interactions of significant others, 60–62

Atypically disfluent stuttering, 88

Auditory behaviors in SIP, 122–123

B

Behavior of parents, potential of to exacerbate or maintain child's stuttering, 24–25

Behavior therapy on preschool treatments for stuttering, influences of, 104

Behavioral diagnosis and identification, 3

Borderline atypically disfluent, 88

C

Caregivers of children who stutter, 35

Child, brief therapy with, 90–92

Child-specific behaviors, 20

Chronic stuttering, 18–19

Classroom, carryover of FRP, implementation, 167–168

Clinic, intervening with child in, 73

Clinical evidence and impressions in SIP, summary of, 125

Communicative environment, modifying, 70

Communicative interactions in parent-child groups, 33–37

Comprehensive therapy program, 92–93

Concepts of FRP, teaching, 166